MW01484201

The
Magical
Sex Book

Also by Wiegers and Claire:

So THAT'S Why They Do That!
Men, Women, And Their Hormones

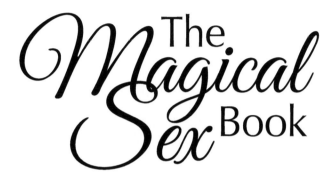

The Magical Sex Book

Create and sustain amazing sex in four simple steps

Frank Wiegers & Judith Claire

The Magical Sex Book
Copyright © 2021 by Frank Wiegers & Judith Claire

All rights reserved. This book or any portion thereof may not be reproduced or used in any manner whatsoever without the express written permission of the publisher except for the use of brief quotations in a book review.

For inquiries, contact:
FrankWiegers
310-337-2701
Frank@themagicalsexbook.com
info@topgunlove.com

Printed in the United States of America

Cover Design: Tatiana Vila, Vila Design
Page Layout: Carla Green, Clarity Designworks

ISBN paperback: 978-0-9911622-0-8
ISBN ebook: 978-0-9911622-1-5
ISBN audio book: 978-0-9911622-2-2

Contents

Preface

I've been passionate about this work for over 35 years, and I'm so excited to share it with you. Sexual fulfillment came late to me because I grew up in a sexually repressed environment. After leaving a passionless marriage in my forties, I had something of a spiritual awakening and began an intensive study of love, sex and relationship. I read every book I could find and studied with teachers from Europe, India, and the U.S., including a Native American shaman. Wow! That opened a whole new world for me.

I always had this sense that sex could be very spiritual, and the more passionate it was, the more spiritual it was. I would get random experiences of "Oh My God" quality sex but couldn't predict when it was going to happen and didn't know how to make it happen on a regular basis.

As I continued my study and training, I was able to get to that place more frequently, but still not on what I would call a sustainable, repeatable experience. Then I met my wife, Judith, and I found I was able to match what I had learned to what she had learned—not just about sex, but about how to communicate and connect, how to treat each other, how to love. It was, and is, magic.

Service is a key value that she and I share. That's why I was a fighter pilot, and why I have coached love, sex, and relationship for 30 years. Judith has been a successful personal, career, and relationship counselor and coach in Los Angeles for over 40 years. We are both dedicated to helping others improve their lives, just as we have improved ours. So, of course, we'd want others to benefit from everything we know about how to create magical sex.

Judith has been my biggest supporter, editor, critic, and not to mention, best lover. She kept reading and suggesting and contributing ideas and pages. I truly appreciate all she did to make this the best book it could be.

I loved writing this book. It kept me turned on about our relationship, our life, and certainly our lovemaking. My deepest wish is that you get as much enjoyment and ecstasy from what's in this book as I did.

Frank

CHAPTER ONE

Introduction: The Quest for Magical Sex

There truly is magic in sex. You know it when it happens — it's when you feel that complete connection to your partner, and you're not sure where you end and they begin. You're both in that mystical place, beyond space and time, and afterward you say something like, "My God. That was amazing!"

Then again, it's not always easy to get to that level of ecstatic transcendence.

If you want that magic on a repeatable and sustainable basis, there are some things you can do to keep that magic in your life. To begin with, there's magic in your deliberate intention to have your love life be magical.

When you know the process, the magic is more likely to occur.

The most important part of the magic comes from the connection to your lover.

So often, couples say that after the first year or so, "the magic went out of their love life." It simply went? Or did they let it go? There is a difference.

We found that those couples started taking their love life for granted and stopped doing all the things that they used to do to make it magical.

A key element in having a lot of that magical sex is having a good, functioning, romantic relationship. The more intimate you are as a couple, the more high levels of ecstasy and fulfillment are available to you. The deeper your connection to your partner, the more likely you are to create a mind-blowingly magical sexual experience.

SEXUAL REVOLUTION TO SEXUAL EVOLUTION

A good start is to learn ways to deepen the level of intimacy, not just sexual intimacy but your intimate connections on all levels. Stop for a minute and remember the beginning of your relationship.

Recall that time when you would do almost anything for your lover.

Think of the caring and nurturing feelings you had back then.

Now think about that level of sensitivity and responsiveness to each other's emotional state that you had, and how you can bring that back.

Look for ways to touch, caress and kiss, whenever and *wherever* possible. That physical connection triggers the release of oxytocin, the bonding hormone, and you will find yourself more deeply in love. When that feeling and connection are carried into the bedroom, the magic happens.

Life, too, happens, and we get caught up in all the things and situations we have to deal with in our lives, losing sight of the thing that matters most to us: our relationship.

On a personal note, I have to tell you this wasn't easy for me either. I was an arrogant fighter pilot who knew it all, and you had to do it my way. The truth was, I knew almost nothing… about sex and relationship.

My biggest concern was scoring and getting my rocks off. I did pick up some techniques that seemed to make some women happy, but I was an amateur.

Sex was important to me, and when relationship after relationship didn't seem to work out, I thought about what the common denominator was, and it was me. So, I started to study and research. I found teachers from all over the world and worked with a shaman for over fifteen years. I read every book I could find, and it seemed like I made some progress. I learned that I had to heal all my old wounds from childhood and other relationships that were getting in my way, and change some false beliefs that were keeping me from having a truly intimate relationship.

IS THIS LIKE TANTRA?

What we teach incorporates many elements of Tantra and many elements of other disciplines as well. So yes, it is somewhat like Tantra, but it isn't classic Tantra.

Then I met my wife, Judith at a Tantric ceremony. In case you didn't know, Tantra is an ancient Hindu or Buddhist teaching involving rituals, yoga, disciplines and meditations. Neo-Tantra is what is most commonly practiced in modern cultures and takes the word Tantra to mean a weaving. In this case, it's a weaving of male/female energy and sexuality into everyday life. Tantra embraces the concept of loving sex as a spiritual practice.

Judith and I clicked immediately and began a relationship that made our sex life a spiritual practice. We were able to use all the studies we each had, and we created the kind of love life I'd always dreamed of.

While it is important to know lovemaking techniques, the real key is in the *connection* on as many levels as possible: physical, emotional, mental, and spiritual. The whole purpose is to create the kind of intimacy that is deep and fulfilling, where you know and feel your partner and your partner knows and feels you, and you trust each other completely. Once the connection is there, then you can use the techniques you know to take it to even higher levels of magical bliss.

FIGHTER PILOTS AND LOVERS

With all that study and practice in the area of sex and relationships, I began to see some parallels to what I had learned and experienced as a fighter pilot. I'll use that comparison all through this book.

Men *may* (although not necessarily) relate to my fighter pilot analogy more than women, unless those women happen to be fighter pilots, so ladies, please do read on. I'm writing as though I'm talking to a guy, but the information is meant for both men and women.

I loved flying jet fighters, almost as much as I loved sex, but flying fighters was dangerous work. We averaged about one crash a month when I was working as an instructor pilot teaching new fighter pilots. You might think that sex and relationships are not as complicated and dangerous as flying a fighter. Think again. At least when you die in a fighter, it's quick.

How you create your sex /love life has a direct bearing on every other aspect of your life. A 2016 study called *Is sex good for your health?* indicated that those who have a satisfying and fulfilling love life perform better in every area, are healthier, and live longer than those who do not. For me personally, when I am verbally and emotionally connected to my lover, and the more connected sex I have, the more creative I am in everything I do.

Those living unconnected, unfulfilled love lives are more likely to encounter illnesses, both physical and emotional. Sex can be a very important part in maintaining a healthy lifestyle.

WHY MEN NEED THIS AND HOW WOMEN CAN COACH THEM

In another 2016 study, *Relationships among marrieds, sexual satisfaction, marital quality and marital instability,* men were asked if they thought they were good lovers. Eighty-five percent of them ranked themselves as "good" to "great" lovers. When their women partners were asked what they thought about their men being good lovers, only fifteen percent of the women agreed with their men.

This tells us two things about men as lovers. First, men really believe they're good at lovemaking, which means they don't know what they don't know, and therefore have no motivation to change or learn something different. Second, their women partners must not have been telling them the truth. Then there are some women who've only had one lover, or a limited number of lovers, and have never had good sex, so they don't know what they're missing.

Perhaps women don't want to bruise men's fragile egos. But for whatever reason, the woman often doesn't tell the man that she's not getting what she wants and needs, so he goes on thinking he's a great lover, and she remains dissatisfied and unfulfilled.

As I began to study and research about having extraordinary sex, I found many similarities between what it takes to be a great lover and what it takes to be a top-gun fighter pilot.

For example, when I was upgrading to a new airplane, or one that was different from the one I had been flying before, I had weeks of special classes that taught me every aspect of how the airplane was put together, how each system worked, and how those systems interfaced with each other. After learning about the airplane, there were classes on procedures and tactics plus hours of simulator training. When the academic phase had reached a certain level, we began to practice these lessons in the airplane, starting with an instructor. Once the instructor felt we were competent enough, we were allowed to do it solo—that is, alone—without supervision.

It was fun and exciting to take those high-performance airplanes and get them to do the things we wanted. Practicing air-to-air combat, dogfighting, was as thrilling as you can imagine. We used to kid each other, saying that the only thing better than flying fighters was having great sex. Having a fulfilling, loving, sexual relationship is the only thing I've found that surpasses the thrill of flying fighters.

What if we had *that* kind of training for love, sex, and relationship?

Read on.

FROM ORDINARY SEX TO AMAZING SEX

I used to think that good sex would happen naturally, especially if I was in love. Anybody can have sex, but having great sex takes study, training, and practice. There might be Sex Ed in schools, but what isn't taught is how to be a great partner and a great lover.

Basic sex, the kind that usually isn't magical, may be instinctive, unlike flying where there isn't much that's natural or instinctive. Everything in flying has to be learned and practiced. Being a great lover also has to be learned and practiced, and like being a great pilot, takes a willingness, courage, and commitment to learn.

To be a great lover means you have to know how your body works and know how your partner's body works, and how they interface. There's more to this than recognizing the obvious body parts. For example, women have a different brain structure than men that allows them to switch from left-to-right brain more easily than men. Women's hormone systems are very different from the hormone systems in men, which provides a whole different set of challenges. All this plays a significant role in our love life, particularly in our sex life.

These gender differences are so basic and so important that Judith and I wrote a book about it, called *So THAT'S Why They Do That! Men, Women, and Their Hormones*. It reveals the ABCs of how men's and women's hormones and brains drive their behavior, thoughts, and feelings. When you understand why gender conflicts arise and have the tools to communicate to resolve them, you can achieve the harmony and joy you deserve. If you are committed to having a great love life, I strongly recommend you read this book.

THEN THERE'S *SEX MAGICK.*

What is that, you ask?

As you may know, thoughts have energy, and what you think about is what you tend to create. The more you think about something, the more energy that thought has, the more you act on it, and the higher the possibility that what you are thinking of will actually show up in your life.

I'm sure you are aware of sexual energy, starting with puberty. You feel it as you get turned on, and it builds as you make love and your passion grows. Very few people, however, consciously use their sexual energy.

Sex Magick harnesses the power of your orgasmic energy and combines it with your thoughts of what you desire. When you think of what it is you want to manifest at or around the time of orgasm, it's like adding booster rockets to your thoughts. When you add the power of the two of you holding the same thought, just after orgasm, magic can happen. For example: closer relationship, radiant health, financial abundance, a new home, career success, a child. On a more altruistic level: peace and harmony, unity in a divisive world, healing for loved ones, social justice, or anything that is dear to your heart.

We'll talk more about this when we get to After-Play in the steps of partner sex.

UNLOCK THE POWER OF THE FOUR STEPS

Let's revisit how flying a fighter may be a good analogy to having a great sexual experience. When we flew a mission, there were four stages:

1. Planning and pre-flight;

2. Take-off and flight to mission area;

3. The mission, and;

4. Return to base and debrief.

Planning involved studying all the elements necessary to accomplish the mission and briefing the pilots. Pre-flight checks make sure the airplane is ready to fly.

Flight to the mission area may require specific routing and formation techniques, as well as navigation frequency and air traffic control frequencies.

All pilots take care to watch for other aircraft. If you haven't been properly briefed, you may not know where to go and what to do.

Once you get to the mission area, you need the skills necessary to complete the mission under what might be difficult circumstances, like somebody shooting at you.

Returning to base is self-explanatory. Once you're back on the ground, debriefing is extremely important so that you can learn whether the objectives were accomplished. Also, each pilot's performance is evaluated, and if mistakes were made, they're analyzed to help that pilot improve their skills.

Similarly, I've identified four stages or steps of partner sex.

As in the flight mission, each step in partner sex plays a vital role, and each one is just as important as the other. If you follow these steps, you'll greatly increase your chances of having a magical and transcendent sexual experience.

These Steps are:

1. Pre-Play

2. Fore-Play

3. The-Play

4. After-Play

In the 1950s, the research team of Masters and Johnson did pioneering work in the area of human sexual response that paved the way for the "sexual revolution" along with the availability of birth control for women. Masters and Johnson were the first to identify four phases of human sexual response.

The phases are:

1. The excitement phase of initial arousal

2. The plateau phase, at full arousal but not yet at orgasm

3. Orgasm

4. The resolution phase, after orgasm

I'll discuss each of these and show you how they fit into the four steps I've identified.

But before we get to that, let's consider a few other mission-critical elements that will help you taxi to the takeoff position.

CREATE A VISION OF YOUR LOVE LIFE

Have you ever given serious thought to the kind of love life you'd like?

What would it take for you to have the magical kind of sex life you want?

Have you discussed it with your partner?

If you want this to work for you, you have to approach it with the same drive and motivation as a top gun fighter pilot. This book has all the procedures and techniques you will need such as how to have fun in Pre-Play, detailed Fore-Play suggestions, and how to get the most out of The-Play and After-Play, to name a few. Study them like a pro and practice those techniques with your partner every chance you get.

Some practices may feel uncomfortable and clumsy at first, but like learning to serve a tennis ball or hit a tee shot on the golf course, it takes training and practice. Let me tell you, I felt really clumsy and a little scared on my first attempt to fly an airplane, to say nothing of my first attempts at partner sex. All this discomfort is only because it's new to you and that's why you and your partner have to be in this together.

Approach this as a learning experiment with promising new experiences that will lead to the greatest sex of your life. When you and your partner are willing to practice all these new things until you get pretty good at them... then really good at them... and eventually master them, your life will change forever.

And there is nothing more fun to master than magical sex.

Ideally, reading this book with your lover might be a good way to cover the necessary topics with minimum embarrassment and maximum impact.

Even if you're flying solo, having this knowledge and these skills will go a long way toward building a great relationship when you meet the one you want.

SEX AS A SPIRITUAL PRACTICE

Once you learn the techniques, you need to practice.

There are two forms of practice. The first reason that you practice is because you want to get better at whatever you're practicing. And you also enjoy the practice. For example, you practice a golf swing by hitting golf balls, which can improve your stroke and be a lot of fun at the same time. Or you play the piano or guitar for the same reasons. This also applies to sex.

The second form of practice is spiritual. If you play golf, or guitar, or cook, or do something else that you love, you might sometimes feel like you're "in the zone." If you pray or meditate, you raise your consciousness and your ability to be present, mindful.

A conscious sexual practice can be both meditative and spiritual, not to mention it's a lot of fun and feels great. If you've ever said, "Oh God, I'm coming," you know you were having a spiritual experience. Magical sex connects me to my partner and takes me beyond this physical plane and into a transcendent dimension.

HOW PRACTICING SEX IS MORE FUN THAN PRACTICING ALMOST ANYTHING ELSE

I remember all the times I neglected the joy of my relationship in favor of work or a hobby. Even today, my biggest obstacles to magical sex are stress and fatigue. If I work too hard, there's no energy for sexual pleasure and recreation. I have to ask myself, "Where are my priorities?" Am I neglecting the things that will actually benefit me the most? It is important to me to set aside time for my relationship. Not just the sex, but time for us to be together and play and enjoy exploring things in nature. Doing those things made my life so much richer. There's much more on this in the next chapter.

Adding in sexual energy kept the fire burning, or at least smoldering. If you want to be sexy, act sexy. That doesn't mean act like a porn performer; it just means keep sex in your thoughts and interactions with your partner. Do only the specific sex acts that you're both comfortable with, intrigued by, excited about. Same with the Sex Magick. If any specific thing in this book raises a red flag in her, or in you for that matter, then set it aside without shame or disappointment.

Take what you like and leave the rest.

CHAPTER TWO

Communication for Lovers

IN TO ME YOU SEE LEADS TO MAGICAL SEX – INTIMACY

Even before we begin a long-term committed relationship, while we are still dating, we strive to make our partners desire us and want to stay with us. We do little things that endear them to us, sometimes big things as well. As the relationship becomes mature and we feel confident they will not leave us, we can get preoccupied with mundane life. All the things we used to do for our partner can get lost in the busyness of living.

When we slow down enough to take a breath, we may realize that we are missing those intimate moments we had with our partner and we would like to have them back, but we're not really sure how to do that.

Just like children, relationships need care and nurturing every day. We manage that with rituals and daily do's.

EASY RITUALS THAT DEEPEN INTIMACY

A ritual is defined as "a way of behaving or a series of actions that people regularly carry out in a particular situation because it is their custom to do so." To revive your loving relationship, it's helpful to make sure you develop rituals that will bring you more intimacy, more joy, and a sense of really being connected to your partner/lover.

Here are some examples of rituals you might want to try:

1. **Getting up and going to bed at the same time**. It's a way of synchronizing your day together. This works great for some people and not others. It's an idea.

2. **Morning worship**. I know this sounds weird, but Judith and I take a few minutes after breakfast and before going to work to do this every day. I tell her that I love her, and then two or three things that I love about her. Then she does the same for me. It's healthy relationship nutrition. It makes us feel good to acknowledge what's right about each other, and it makes us feel seen, close, and loved. After doing this for a while it becomes repetitive, but that doesn't matter. It's just the idea that we are taking the time to adore and validate each other.

3. **Mid-day check-in**. My father did this one religiously. He would call my mother every day after lunch just to say hello and tell her he loved her. A modern-day version of this could be sending a text, but don't short-change the moment. Choose a way to communicate that tells the other person you value them.

4. **The evening news**. We usually do this at the dinner table, when we tell each other in detail about what we did that day, who we talked to, how we felt, where we went and anything else of interest. This is important for guys to understand. The idea here is that you are keeping open communication lines with your partner. By conversing with her, you are deepening the bond and the love between you. Tell your partner everything that's going on at work: what you accomplished; what you are having trouble with; and anything at all that's happening there. Then listen with interest as she describes her day and ask questions as appropriate.

5. **Once we are in bed for the night** and before we go to sleep, we tell each other three things:

   a. Things we are grateful for that day. I think gratitude should be on every list of relationship rituals because it maintains your perspective and reminds you how fortunate you are.

The next two items are personal to us. We decided that there were things we wanted to remind ourselves of, and this would highlight them.

    b. We tell each other something we liked about ourselves that day. This takes our attention off of being self-critical and puts it on being self-loving. Much better.

    c. We share what we did for fun that day. We can get lost in work, so this makes us accountable for doing something fun every day.

You can customize this pre-sleep ritual for your own needs. It's a loving way to feel good about your day and create intimacy.

6. **Remember special days**. Don't miss a birthday or anniversary. Be sure they're in your digital calendar. Adding a little gift, not expensive but enough to show you gave it some thought, is a huge bonus.

DAILY DO'S

These next six items are verbal and non-verbal ways of communicating your love for each other. We do them all as often as possible.

1. **Touching**. We never pass by each other without some kind of touch. If she's sitting at the table and I walk by, I'll run my fingers across her shoulders or her back. If we're both in the kitchen, we'll deliberately bump into each other, or grab a quick kiss.

2. **Talking**. Telling her often how I love her and how beautiful she is, thanking her for something she did that was above and beyond the call of duty.

3. **Spending focused time together**. Date nights, walks in the park, mini-getaways, all help fuel the flame of devotion and connection.

4. **Stoking the fire**. Sometimes, at any time of the day, without any intention of having sexual intercourse, we'll kiss and touch or stroke each other just enough to be a turn-on. Maybe we'll do it just for a minute or two, or a little longer, then stop and go about whatever we were doing.

5. **Lightening the load.** Any little chore you can do that will make your partner's life easier and less stressful will go a long way toward endearment.

6. **Snuggling.** Many times when we're in bed with the lights out, I snuggle up behind her, feeling her body against mine. It's such a warm, comforting place to be and sleep comes quickly. Sometimes she will snuggle up to me and put her arms around me and onto my chest or stomach and we'll fall asleep that way. This works if either of us wakes at night or in the early hours of the morning, we often snuggle and we both go back to sleep very quickly.

These are all suggestions and you can modify them and use them however you like.

The idea is to do some of these things on a regular basis so you nurture your relationship. Relationships need care and attention on a daily basis. These rituals will help with that process. The payoff is deeper intimacy and a strong relationship that will lead you to higher levels of love and bliss and stronger support in times of need. When you get so in-tune with each other, you know what the other person is going to say before they say it, you communicate with knowing looks, and you feel that vibe when you look at her, knowing how much you love her.

LIMBIC RESONANCE

Once you develop and sustain this loving connection, you will experience a phenomenon called "limbic resonance," which is a deep empathy, almost a psychic connection with your partner. You "vibe" together, "feel" together, and "resonate" together.

There is an area of the brain called the limbic lobe. It releases certain chemicals that are vital to our emotional and physical well-being. When two people interact in a safe, loving relationship, they stimulate these brain chemicals.

Here's what Wikipedia has to say about that:

> *Limbic resonance is the idea that the capacity for sharing deep emotional states arises from the limbic system of the brain. These states include the dopamine circuit-promoted feelings of empathic harmony, and the norepinephrine circuit-originated emotional states of fear, anxiety and anger.*

> The concept was advanced in the book, *A General Theory of Love* (2000) and is one of three interrelated concepts central to the book's premise that our brain chemistry and nervous systems are measurably affected by those closest to us (limbic resonance); that our systems synchronize with one another in a way that has profound implications for personality and lifelong emotional health (limbic regulation);

and that these set patterns can be modified through therapeutic practice (limbic revision).

In other words, it refers to the capacity for empathy and non-verbal connection that is present in mammals, and that forms the basis of our social connections as well as the foundation for various modes of therapy and healing.

According to the authors our nervous systems are not self-contained, but rather demonstrably attuned to those around us with whom we share a close connection:

"Within the effulgence of their new brain, mammals developed a capacity we call 'limbic resonance' — a symphony of mutual exchange and internal adaptation whereby two mammals become attuned to each other's inner states."

Limbic resonance is one of the great joys of magical sex. To get to that magical place, we have to tell our partners how we like to be made love to. We have to coach our partners in how to romance and seduce us. So, why do so many of us fail to communicate our needs to each other?

There are lots of reasons. Some men and women are too inhibited or shy to speak up; others are afraid to be rejected; some guys are arrogant and think they know it all.

By far the main problem is that so many women are hesitant to tell their lovers what works personally for them. They are afraid of the consequences of bruising the infamous male ego. Their fear is well-founded. Men often take any comments about sexual performance as criticism, and it shuts them down.

For many men, being told that they're not doing something right during sex is like an affront to their masculinity. It's as if they don't measure up or aren't good enough.

This is a very sensitive area. The truth is that most men have never really had the necessary training to be a good lover or, just as important, to do well in an intimate relationship with a woman.

I was one of those guys.

HOW TO GET WHAT YOU WANT IN THE BEDROOM

First you have to know what you're working with.

HOW SOME MEN ARE

Remember the study I mentioned, where men think they are great lovers, but their women don't necessarily agree with them?

Well, guys, you have to know it's hard for women to talk to us about their sexual needs. They've probably been rebuffed so many times that they're a little gun-shy. You have to actually encourage her to tell you what she wants, and you also need to genuinely want to hear her answers. This isn't just going through the motions.

If you want magical sex, you must be open to learning what she wants and then giving her what she asks for.

What I hear from a lot of women is that men just do what they want without any regard for what the woman wants. For example: shoving her head down to his crotch without asking, slamming into her deep and hard without preparation, deep tongue kissing without caring about her sensibilities: it's a long list.

If a man received any sexual training at all, it was probably a combination of Sex Ed class in school, an occasional Playboy article, and what he learned from his buddies or his father, most of which is not helpful for our purposes.

The sex presented in the porno videos today has very little to do with having a real, fulfilling sexual relationship with a real live woman. In fact, a lot of porn is so misleading that it actually inhibits having connected, magical sex.

We men are a funny lot. We'll spend countless dollars and countless hours on our hobby. We hire pros, coaches, and trainers. However, when it comes to listening to the woman in our life trying to teach us how she wants us to make love to her, we resist and ignore her advice.

It's time to tamp down our male egos and listen to what she says.

The information I gleaned in talking to my friends about how to please a woman sexually was usually incomplete and often wrong. I was too embarrassed to ask specific questions of my friends because I really didn't even know what questions to ask. I also thought that because one woman I'd been making love with liked what I was doing, that technique should work on a different woman as well. Wrong.

HOW SOME WOMEN ARE

It's essential for both men and women to take responsibility for what they want. You have to help her to be clear about what she wants and to take action toward getting it.

I hear from some women that they don't want to have to "train" their lover. He should come to the relationship already perfectly attuned to their woman's sexual appetites. Sorry to say that, realistically, a large percentage of men are both ignorant and apathetic. They don't know what their women want, and they don't care.

I understand it's challenging for a lot of women to ask for what they want sexually. Here's the thing ladies: he won't know what you want unless you tell him, out loud, in words. It will relieve a lot of stress and tension for him if he knows what you want. He may just be doing what he thinks will make you happy.

WHAT WOMEN NEED TO LEARN

Women have to ask for what they want in a way that a man can hear and understand, while men need to hear what women want, out loud, in words, and probably more than once. This can be difficult for many women who are natural receivers and not inclined to ask.

That's why it might work better to have these kinds of conversations in some place other than the bedroom during sex. But please don't do it while he's driving or occupied with something else. Make sure you have his full attention.

Some women do speak up in sex, however, the way they speak up is counter-productive.

For me, communicating about sex used to be awkward and embarrassing, especially while in the act of making love. A lover would say something like, "Don't do that!" or "That hurts!" and I would take her comment as a criticism of my lovemaking skills and feel wounded and offended. This would cause me to lose interest, lose my erection, or get mad at her. All she was trying to do was tell me what to avoid so that she would enjoy it as much as I was enjoying it. Eventually, she stopped trying, because it was fruitless and she didn't want me to feel inadequate.

Sex partners often told me what *not* to do, but rarely gave me any friendly guidance on what I *should* be doing.

For example, there may be times when a woman sees her lover is struggling to get her to orgasm, and all she wants is that afterglow connection with him, she has to let him know not to keep pounding away, or licking away as the case might be.

WHAT MEN NEED TO LEARN

If a woman is having trouble verbalizing her needs, try to help her be clear by creating a safe space for her. When she does tell you what she wants, you can't debate or argue with her. She's telling you what would make her happy. It's her perception, not yours, so just listen, acknowledge what she says, and keep asking her if there's any more she needs to tell you.

In fact, keep asking, "Is there more?" until she's said it all.

Whatever you do, don't judge or criticize anything she says.

If she doesn't know what to ask for, tell her you want to keep reading this book together and see what it brings up. You can use the list in Appendix III and ask her what she thinks about each item on the list.

Remember, if you don't ask, the answer is always, "No."

The only way to get past our wrong assumptions about one another's sexual curiosities and desires is through effective communication.

Men have to be open and willing to listen and change.

Every woman has different neural pathways in her pelvic area. No two women are exactly alike, so doing the same thing with every woman is not going to lead to orgasm for each one.

You learn, you listen, you care enough to serve your lover's needs, and you're humble and authentic enough to understand her so that she has the greatest pleasure possible.

Every woman I talked with also agreed that she had to learn new ways to please each man. Making love is specific to who you are making love with. It takes communication and practice to reach that place of magical sex.

CREATE A LOVING CONVERSATION ABOUT LOVING SEX

The first thing is to set a time and place to have non-judgmental, non-antagonistic discussions about what you want and how to get it from the other person. It's better to have these talks outside the bedroom. What works really well is to have them while taking a walk together. That way, she gets to go for a walk with you, and she gets a conversation, which bonds her to you. Plus, by the end of your walk, you both will have a better understanding of what each of you wants in the bedroom.

Another approach is to sit in a comfortable private place so you won't be disturbed. Have some coffee or tea or even a glass of wine, but don't overdo it with the alcohol.

You can start by asking each other to share two or three things you each like about your sex life. Then describe two or three things you could do to improve your sex life, the old "what works and what doesn't work?" analysis. To allay her fears of inadequacy (we all have them!), you could phrase it as "what is great about our sexual relationship, and what might make it even better." Then brainstorm, in a cooperative way, to find things you can both do to make your sex life better.

These conversations can go a long way in enabling you and your lover how to communicate about sex and get what you each need. This also helps to bust through some old inhibiting beliefs and launch a new, improved sex life. The key element for men is, be teachable!

GOING DEEPER

You both need to agree that the main goal: to *teach each other how to be better lovers for each other*. Men also need to agree not to get offended or hostile when getting directions. You need to follow her guidance. Be curious about what she has to say because it's important to her and to you as well. Don't judge her. Be positive and open. This is about creating intimacy, which will give you the hottest sex ever.

LADIES FIRST

Begin by asking her these three questions:

1. Is there anything I could do to improve your comfort, or make you more comfortable? If she says yes, discuss what alternatives you have. You may have to experiment.

2. Do I do anything that you don't like? Or that you'd rather I not do? Ask her why she would rather not do those things and accept her answers without arguing.

If there's a deeper answer, she'll tell you later. For instance, she might say at first that she doesn't like fellatio (blow jobs) because "it's kinda gross," but later she may confess a traumatic experience that could be healed together with you in a completely different atmosphere of delight—or you both might just seal up that trauma in the past and explore other ways of pleasuring one another. So your next question would be...

3. Is there anything particular you would like me to do?

After she's answered, it's her turn to ask you the same questions. Make it clear that she can revisit these questions anytime she likes!

IN BED

Once you're in the throes of passion, women need to let your partner know what is working or if anything hurts or simply doesn't feel good. Express it as politely as possible.

Guys, this is a time and place where paying close attention is extremely important.

You can't phone this in.

If some activity can be improved, tell him it feels wonderful, but suggest a variation such as "Would you mind doing it (harder/ softer), (higher/lower), more to the (right/left) (up/down)." Thank them for making the change. "Oh yeah, that feels so much better."

One woman told me that her partner was extremely sensitive to what she said; she had to be very careful. She would approach redirection gently and managed to flatter him at the same time!

She'd say something like, "I don't know if you noticed but you just did X and then Y! It was amazing!"

He would think—oh, did I?

And then he would do it "again" even if he had never done that exact thing before. So, for example, if he finally found the perfect spot on the clitoris, she would say, "When you touched me just there, it was so good." This way, he believed he did something by accident and it worked. It avoided having to tell him to change the tactic as he believed he had done it anyway and just needed to remember it.

She would also say, "I bet you'd really be amazing at X and Y!"

He needed that confidence boost to know she had faith in him to do the right thing and do it well. Then he could pursue her pleasure in the best possible ways, which is the goal for each partner in this process.

Repeat the process until you both get exactly what you want. That way you're cooperating with each other the whole time.

If something is fabulous and you don't want them to stop, or want to intensify the sensation, you can say:

- That's fantastic! Don't stop!

- Oh, do it (harder/softer), (higher/lower), more to the (right/left) (up/down).

- Thank you!

Another example might sound like this: "I love it when you stroke my thigh. Would you do it a little softer?" Sometimes, just a moan or a sigh of delight, or an "Oh, yeah," is enough of a clue to let your partner know they are doing something right. This is an ongoing process.

Oh, and just because your lover says she likes it a certain way on one day, doesn't mean it will be the same the next day. Especially for younger women. Their sensitivity can be so affected by hormone cycles that you have to be prepared to monitor her responses every time. By that I mean, does it look like she's enjoying what you are doing? Some women on certain kinds of birth control may not be experiencing a menstrual cycle, and her sensitivity may not change all that much. Ask about that.

Is she making pleasurable noises, moans, sighs, etc.? If she's just lying there inert, maybe stop and ask if what you're doing feels good or would she rather you do something else?

You can learn how she likes to have her clitoris stimulated if she is willing to show you. She can touch herself while you watch, or she can put her hand over yours while you touch her.

That way, she can direct you to just the right place and just the right pressure.

Some women like a feather light touch and others prefer a firmer, harder touch. Some women even like having their pussy spanked. Most men rarely guess right, so if she wants a good job from you, she has to coach you. It takes patience and repetition, using that three-step process. So put your ego aside and *be teachable*.

If she's adventurous, you might ask her to describe a really good masturbation experience and then have her do that. If she's too shy or uncomfortable with doing that, don't belabor it. If she's open and willing and does it, watch her carefully and learn how she does what gets her the most aroused, and how she reached her orgasm.

If she's struggling to tell you, try sharing your own best masturbation experiences, and then she may be more reassured into sharing hers.

EXCHANGING IDEAS

Tell her some things you like to do and ask her what she thinks about that. Then ask her if there is anything special she likes and see what she says. Remember that and do what she described when the time is right.

On the other hand, some women, because of their background, really don't know what they want. No matter how you ask, they honestly cannot say. I have been able to make some women happy by showing them things I had learned in the past. Another approach I used was to get books and sex manuals about things I wanted to try, then she and I would read them together and try different techniques. You can do that with this book. It's a great thing to do to keep variety in your sex life and it brings you closer. Sharing something so intimate—possibly things that nobody else even knows—will draw you together.

It's very important for women to know that they have to communicate, out loud, in words, to their man. You need to tell her that it's not only fine to say what she wants, but necessary. She needs to know that it won't be a turn-off for you. She needs to say whether what you're doing is turning her on or not.

To the woman reading this: if you are too turned on to talk, make sounds, happy moans, an "Oh yeah," or "Don't stop," and he will love you for "You are *so* good at that."

You may not realize this, but men also need reassurance and encouragement, and this alone will help your man to improve his techniques. Giving him confidence means he'll not be afraid to try things out, and if you tell him how much you love certain things, he will not be so disappointed or affronted if the occasional thing does not work for you so well.

The real key to magical sex is your connection to your partner, and one of the ways to establish and strengthen your connection to your partner is by using the rituals and daily do's I described earlier and the rituals around sex that are to come in the following chapters.

ROI

So, what's the payoff for all the time and effort required to get her to a super-sizzling, magical orgasm?

It's huge.

She will feel so energized and enlivened that her energy will flow to you and you will be empowered by it. This energy is healing and creative, and you will want as much of it as you can get. Taking the time to bring her to this open, trusting, and relaxed space will have a similar effect on you, and your orgasm will be more powerful and fulfilling. Your connection to her will be deeper and more sexually charged.

That's why Pre-Play is so important.

This is not to say that every time you make love, it has to be a two-to-three-hour event. However, if you don't do this regularly, you are leaving a lot of wonderful healing and creative energy on the table.

CHAPTER THREE

Male Orgasm Training

MULTIPLE ORGASMS AND PROLONGING ORGASM FOR MEN

Why men's orgasm training? Well, because I've noticed in recent years that many of the women's magazines have tips on how women can have deeper orgasms, longer orgasms, nipple orgasms, anal orgasms, cervical orgasms, and all manner of techniques for getting there.

Yet I haven't ever seen that kind of attention for men.

Many men aren't even aware that they can have multiple orgasms or non-ejaculatory orgasms, or that they can be made to ejaculate with prostate massage—which, by the way, doesn't give you the same feeling you get with your usual orgasm.

Many of us men grew up masturbating quietly and quickly to relieve that pressure that drove us crazy. If we didn't have a room of our own, we had to do it in the bathroom or the shower, having had no other personal space where we could do it undisturbed. Even if we did have a room, we often were worried that someone could walk in on us and we be embarrassed.

As a result, we trained ourselves to orgasm in the fastest way possible, and for some men, this led to having premature ejaculations when having partner sex. This is not the kind of sexual experience we want to have now. We need training and practice to reprogram those muscle memories and our emotional approach as well.

ORGASM TRAINING

Here are a few suggestions for how to do that.

First of all, many men masturbate on a regular basis, whether they're in a relationship or not. Those in a relationship may feel that they are taking the pressure off their women partners by not demanding sex every time they feel the urge. There's no shame or stigma to masturbating, it's just something you can do. On the other hand, if you are masturbating to the point that you are neglecting your partner, that's not a good thing.

You can use masturbation to learn new techniques to control your orgasm and actually gain energy while doing it.

Here's what to do:

1. Plan to allow at least thirty minutes for this practice.

2. Get yourself set up with whatever lube you use, and any porn or visual stimulus you might need.

3. Once you begin, stroke yourself to the point that if you continue, you will orgasm.

4. Stop at least two strokes short of an ejaculatory orgasm.

When you are at that point, stop all stimulation, take a full deep breath and clench your PC muscles (that's the muscle you use to stop peeing). Hold the PC clench and then visualize all the energy you have in your genitals (you can think of that energy as a soft warm sphere) and bring it up your spinal column, all the way to your heart.

Once your need to orgasm has subsided, begin to stimulate yourself again. Bring yourself right to the edge of orgasm and again, stop stimulation, take a deep inhale as you clench your PC muscle, and bring all the sexual energy up into your heart. If you like, you can bring that energy up to your brain as well.

Bring yourself to that edge just before orgasm at least six times in a thirty-minute period. At the end of the exercise, you can go to a full ejaculation or save that energy for when you are with your partner. This practice is commonly called "edging."

You can use this energy to empower your creativity and the love you share in the world.

You can also do Sex Magick with this energy, just as you would in partner sex. For a more detailed description, see the section in Chapter Seven on Sex Magick.

PREMATURE EJACULATION (PE)

Some men get very stressed out about ejaculating before they want to, and before the woman has had any satisfaction at all. The more they think and worry about PE, the worse it gets, and this can often ruin the whole sexual experience. If you ejaculate before you want to, it doesn't mean that you have to stop making love.

That's not necessarily the end of it, because 50-80 percent of women don't orgasm during intercourse. So you can bring her to orgasm manually or orally or both, and maybe in that process, your erection might return and you can have another chance. Using the orgasm training should help as well. It's always a good idea to bring her to orgasm first in any case.

Some women have said that they find very gratifying when a man orgasms quickly with her. She has him so hot and bothered he can't hold back. She may not want a prolonged effort to bring him to orgasm, or to bring her to orgasm every time. Quick and furtive sex can be passionate and fulfilling, and can be magical as well, for both partners.

Even when PE is not an issue, men often suffer from performance anxiety. They want to make a good impression on a woman who is a new lover and get so nervous they lose their erection. Take a pill, for God's sake.

Generic forms of Cialis, Viagra, and all the rest, are widely and discreetly available. Take the pressure off yourself so you can relax and give her the kind of sex she wants to get from you. You'll have a better time too.

CHAPTER FOUR

Step 1: Pre-Play

WHAT IS PRE-PLAY?

The purpose of Pre-Play is to set the context and get you both completely present in the moment, opening the door for a powerful connection between the two of you. The context includes where you are, who you're with, what you're doing, and what's going on in your head.

This first step, to "pre-heat the romance," is the least understood, and the most neglected. Yet it is profoundly important in the process of achieving magical sex. Everything that follows will build upon whatever you do at this step. With Pre-Play, you are building a stable foundation for your sexual connection, so that Fore-Play will be so much better, and The-Play will reach mind-blowing heights. The depth of your connection will determine the heat of the sizzle. The hotter the sizzle, the more powerful the magic.

If you skip this step, the odds of getting to magical sex are much lower. Actually, you may not get to sex at all. Pre-Play can defuse a whole bunch of excuses like "too tired, headache," and so on.

Here are some things to consider about Pre-Play and then some techniques you can actually use during Pre-Play. Keep in mind that Pre-Play is PLAY. Make it fun; it's a form of romance and seduction.

BEFORE PRE-PLAY

There are elements of Pre-Play that take place outside the bedroom and before the date and time of your tryst. These are the things we talked about in Chapter 2, using the rituals and developing limbic resonance.

DATE NIGHT

Pre-play can also be dinner and a movie. Date night is really important, or a date day if you can manage it. Something that gets you out of your usual space and creates a sense of adventure. It could be a sporting event, a museum, or some kind of performing art. Sometimes a walk in the local park may be just what it takes.

Pre-play can be different every time. Sometimes, you are both so horny that you just kiss and tear each other's clothes off and get it on! That sort of urgency can be a powerful kind of "instant Pre-Play" as long as both partners are feeling it.

CALENDAR SEX

For those who are in a well-established long-term committed relationship, it's a good idea to calendar your time for sex. I can hear the women saying, "But that's not spontaneous." That is true. But the time when you could rely on "just tear our clothes off and get it on!" probably passed after your first couple of years of being together.

Calendaring romance and sex is especially important for those in long-term relationships, where your desire for each other fluctuates. Desire is good; however, when desire isn't strong, just showing up will get things started, and the end result is usually very good. Pre-Play will you put into the right frame of mind. Knowing that great sex is important enough for your partner to put in the calendar, protecting it from the demands and distractions of life, can be a Pre-Play turn-on all its own.

In many cases, there may not even be a desire for sex until things actually get started, and you both become aroused. Desire will follow arousal.

I always thought that I needed to feel some sexual desire *before* I could get in the mood to have sex. What I learned was that if I got started, just fooling around acting sexual, I would get turned on, and then the desire was there.

Judith tells me the same thing works for her.

So, the secret is, make the time and space to have sex, get naked and start playing, and fun and magic may follow. It's the old truth in action: "suit up and show up, and the game is on."

That's why it's a good idea to have calendared sex. It's a good opportunity to make things special. Scheduling sex may not seem spontaneous and in-the-moment; however, the *kind* of sex you have can be very spontaneous. And just because you have scheduled sex doesn't mean you cannot have *unscheduled* sex whenever the mood grabs you. In fact, scheduled sex may be what you need to get feeling sexy again—it could lead to lots of other surprises!

The idea is that you both know you are creating the time and space to have that all important sexual connection that will keep your relationship strong and thriving.

DESIRE FOLLOWS AROUSAL

If you get together in bed, naked, and just touch each other and feel the connection, oxytocin, the bonding hormone, will start to flow and arousal happens. Once you're aroused, you feel the insistent urge of desire.

Make yourself present with the intention of having a good sexual experience and then let it happen. The messages you tell yourself are also important, so be sure to use plenty of positive affirmation, such as.

I can't wait for our intimacy night!

God, I feel so sexy today.

We are going to enjoy great lovemaking.

Avoid getting lost in the *what-ifs* and don't worry about it if it doesn't always happen when planned. That's life.

But if it does—or rather, *when* it does!—go with it. Let it happen and flow.

The last thing we want is routine sex, so feel free to spice it up a little if that's what works for you. Pick your venue carefully and think of where you had the best, most fun, most engaging and close sex previously, or whatever works for both of you.

Just a note here. Some couples say they "only" have bedroom sex. As if sex in a bedroom is inherently boring. That is really downplaying the magic that can happen in the bedroom! Or any room!

SETTING THE SCENE

Using the bedroom doesn't mean the sex has to be routine just because that's where you usually make love. Take some time to make it special.

Of course, in the bedroom, pick up any clutter, straighten the sheets and pillows, set the lighting, use incense, buy some special drinks, treat her to new lingerie—yes, guys, this means *you too.* Not even your wife wants to see those saggy undershorts or holey socks—and do whatever else you can to make it sensual and inviting.

You can even agree to buy each other a 'special something' for that night. Keep it small and inexpensive, a token of your special night and something really fun you can laugh about.

ONE EXAMPLE

Here's how one woman told me she likes to set up her bedroom before having sex.

> "I use two smaller firm pillows on either side of my partner when I'm on top and straddling him. This helps in several ways: Because I'm smaller, it lifts me up several inches so that I can fully move more comfortably (and accommodate his long cock) when fucking him. These pillows also save my knees. Since I'm short and my partner is wider than I am, having these 'props' handy really keeps the sex flowing comfortably and I can maintain my position longer.
>
> "Also, when I'm on my back with my legs spread, placing a pillow under each thigh (behind the knee) helps to keep my back supported and comfortable. I can fuck longer with this simple technique.
>
> "I find it's good to keep an array of pillows of varying sizes handy for when I need a bit more comfort or support. One more thing... if a lover

is using a dildo to pleasure me (and yes, I enjoy my array of toys), I want to make sure it's warm. There's nothing worse than having a cold, hard device entering you! I have a small heating pad on which I place my toys and then cover them with a towel to keep them vagina-ready. I keep my lube on the pad too. Coconut oil is our go-to lube."

I like her ideas and we use pillows for comfort as well.

SEX MAGICK CEREMONY PREPARATION

If you are planning to do a special 'Sex Magick Ceremony' after your orgasms, you must declare your intentions and make sure everything you want is set up. For more details on how to do this, see Step 4 in Chapter Seven.

You might choose somewhere else besides the bedroom, but if it is to be bedroom sex, well, why not? Just make it special. There are many options. If one of you is less than comfortable with a certain place, just avoid that and go for what meets both of your needs.

Also, try to think of it like you're going to a special event. You would dress well and would act respectfully in the environment. Go to your bedroom with that kind of idea. Be freshly showered and smell nice. Look your best. Wear something sexy, or at least attractive. After all, you are going to a spiritual service.

GETTING IN TUNE FOR MAGICAL SEX

In order for a woman to have magical sex:

- She must feel *safe,*

- She must feel *relaxed* and

- She must feel *lovingly connected.*

In many cases, even if a woman doesn't feel all of these things, and feels some stress, she may be able to get aroused and even have an orgasm. However, it may not have the power of a *magical, sizzling* orgasm. If she feels criticized or belittled in any way, she won't feel safe.

If she feels cold or in any way uncomfortable, she won't be fully relaxed. If her feet are chilly, it may be just enough distraction to keep her from having that magical experience. Encourage her to put on some socks, in that case. No big deal. If she doesn't feel you are fully present and lovingly interested in bringing her to the ultimate bliss, she will not feel connected.

If your goal is to have magical sex, it's worth the time and effort to help her release her stress, and then she can be totally present and enjoy herself. You will also enjoy it more too.

VERBAL COMMUNICATION

Getting into communication is the very start of Pre-Play.

To be sure I'm making myself clear, I want to say again that:

The foundation for MAGICAL SEX is in the CONNECTION and the way to CONNECTION is COMMUNICATION.

For most women, talking is *the* way to get into connection.

When women talk, they generate oxytocin, the bonding hormone, plus dopamine and norepinephrine, a real chemical cocktail. The more they talk, the more oxytocin, dopamine, and norepinephrine they release, the deeper the bond and the better, more connected they feel. This is a major component in achieving magical sex.

In communication, each person is expressing their thoughts, ideas, problems, joys and creativity. If you aren't judgmental and create a safe space, you can have the privilege of seeing your lover's internal life and vice versa. Being non-judgmental is also being tolerant. Journeying into each other's world can make you see what you agree with and like, which makes you closer. This is real intimacy.

If she brings up a problem about something in her life (other than about the relationship), this is not the time for you to play "Mr. Fix-It." Many times when a woman is talking about a situation or an issue, she is only exploring it to understand if it really is a problem or not. It doesn't need "fixing."

Listen, so she feels heard. Empathize.

Get her talking about other things too. Ask her a few questions and let her talk. Ask her what her plans are, what clothes she's thinking about, what shows she wants to watch, what she's working on.

Listen to her and stay engaged. You might think it sounds trite, but the point is that you show you are interested in *her,* and this will excite and please her. Although romantic words and caresses are the spark that starts the flame, plain conversation may not be merely a great prelude to foreplay—it may be the foreplay she desires the most.

NON-VERBAL COMMUNICATION

Talking is just one way that we get into communication.

There are many non-verbal ways of communicating: a smile or a frown, body language, eye gazing, and synchronized breathing are all ways that we can communicate with each other. Throughout the practice, *smile* at each other. This tells your brain that you are happy, which will subconsciously elevate your mood. It also tells your partner you're happy to be with her.

The idea is that we want that deep connection, and communication in many forms is the way to achieve it and retain it. When the connection is strong, you feel the power of it.

The bond between the two of you creates a powerful spiritual presence that becomes another element. There's *you*, and there's *her*, and there's the *relationship*.

This is the real holy trinity that leads to transcendence, that experience that takes us above and beyond our normal plane of awareness.

GO, SLOW, OR STOP?

Before you start, ask yourselves if you have a red light, yellow light, or green light as you are moving toward your tryst.

If it's green, full speed ahead.

If it's yellow, take a look at what might be slowing you down and see what you can do to remove anything that could be blocking you from having a magical sexual encounter. This might be something as simple as clearing off a cluttered workspace (often the kitchen table) together, affirming, "This is all important and none of it will be forgotten. But we are done for now. We'll deal with this tomorrow." It might be a physical issue like a tension headache, back pain, or foot pain: taking steps to alleviate that pain, simply out of loving concern, can change the yellow light to green. Or it might require clearing up a bit of relational friction between you: a face-to-face apology might be enough, or it might require a longer conversation. Any degree of resolution is better than none, and may turn the light green.

Or it may reveal that it was a red light all along.

If it's red, then stop. If there are issues that will keep you from being completely present in the moment and lovingly engaged with your partner, then any sexual experience might be the opposite of magical; it might end up frustrating or unfulfilling.

Do your best to clear up these issues before you start.

If she does bring up an issue with you that is unresolved, it's a tricky situation. On one hand, that issue may inhibit her participation and block any chance for an ecstatic, magical sexual experience.

On the other hand, it may trigger a hot button and lead to a long processing session. If that's the case, it's better to stop and resolve the issue and then have make-up sex afterward. This also sets you up for a greater depth of communication and closeness—and even more fantastic sex down the line as your relationship gets even stronger.

If she is feeling stressed, that's going to inhibit her ability to have magical sex anyway (and the same for you), so you need to go into it with matters resolved.

FOR WOMEN

Just as there are many ways a woman likes to be seduced, so it is for men too.

Most men love it when their woman initiates sex.

Men are also very visual. Many respond positively to costumes or sexy lingerie. Some examples are a baby-doll or a teddy, a sexy nurse's uniform, a sexy school-girl uniform with a pleated skirt and knee-high socks. The classic thigh-high stockings with garter belt, shelf bra, and spike heels is always a killer. Ask him what kind of lingerie or costume he might like, and if it isn't a turnoff for you, experiment with that.

Making eye contact while flirting or talking sexy, sharing fantasies, teasing and tempting, are all great "come-ons." Fixing him a drink and telling him what you want to do and how you want to do it always works well.

Planning a honeymoon getaway can get the creative and romantic juices flowing, even if the trip itself may be a fantasy.

Touching, body massage, foot massage, rubbing him all over with your hands and nails, running your hands through his hair, licking or blowing softly into his ear, grabbing his butt or his balls are other good ploys. Playing with him under the table in a restaurant can be very exciting. Taking him to a sex-toy store and talking about how you would use the toys can be a turn on.

Kiss him. French kiss him. Surprise him with a passionate kiss in the car or some other unusual place.

WHAT TO DO DURING PRE-PLAY

Now let's talk about the Pre-Play that takes place in the bedroom or wherever it is you're going to make love.

You've set a date and time to meet in the bedroom or wherever you've agreed upon.

Before the agreed time, you've taken showers or freshened up. Tidy up the room and make sure the temperature is comfortable. If you're going to do a ceremony, set that up.

Get together on the bed (or wherever you might be) facing each other in the nude, and talk until you feel you are in communication with each other.

A VERY IMPORTANT PART

Once you feel connected, go to Appendix II and do the movement and sitting exercises we've listed there. We've found them to intensify our sexual experience both physically and spiritually.

Sometimes when we feel tired, distracted, or time constrained, we've skipped the exercises and gone straight into Fore-Play. The result almost always is a lower energy level, especially on the spiritual connection, and the level of magic we reach is not as high as we want.

Another plus is that many of these exercises are basic tools that you can use during sex, adding an exciting new dimension to your lovemaking.

So, if you really want magical sex, do these exercises.

CHAPTER FIVE

Step 2: Fore-Play

FANNING THE FLAMES OF AROUSAL TO CREATE DESIRE

So now you've done enough Pre-Play to establish a nice, warm, intimate connection. The next step is to create arousal which will stoke the flames of desire. That's the real purpose of Fore-Play. The focus in Fore-Play is on the woman, since men don't usually need a lot of foreplay. What men need usually is to be seduced, and that is part of Pre-Play.

Once a woman feels the connection, her oxytocin is flowing, and she is feeling bonded. She's not yet at arousal. The Pre-Play opens the door to arousal a lot wider.

The processes and techniques of Fore-Play require some skill and understanding. Most guys usually know by now not to go straight for her erogenous zones, since that is not the best way to get her aroused. She has to get present in her body first, and the way to make that happen is to touch her everywhere *but* her erogenous zones. That means about ten to fifteen minutes of stroking all over her body.

KISSING

One of the most intimate things we can do with another person is kiss them. There are many references to the fact that sex workers may have sex with another person, but they won't kiss them because it's too intimate. So before you go jamming your tongue down her throat, it is a good idea to find out if she's ready for that or even wants it. Kissing a woman the wrong way or at the wrong time can slow down the arousal process and even completely inhibit the whole sexual experience.

Kissing is a great topic for discussion other than in the moment. Take the time to ask her how she likes to be kissed. Most guys just blast ahead and get it wrong. I can remember being taken aback when a woman I had been kissing told me she didn't like deep tongue kissing, and all the while I was getting turned on by what I was doing. If you're not sure, ask.

If you are in the moment, you can put your lips gently on hers and see how she responds. Then mimic what she does and take it soft and slow.

FORE-PLAY SCENARIO

It might look something like this:

You have finished Pre-Play and are lying on the bed, naked. She is lying on her back and you are lying alongside her, on your side, propped up on an elbow, looking at her. Remember, you want to awaken her whole body before you get to the erogenous zones. Start by stroking her arms with a feather light touch. Pay particular attention to the inside of her elbows, and her wrists.

If she is ready for kissing, then kiss her while you are stroking her. Keep the stroking going along her sides and down her stomach, to her legs. Tease her legs open a bit so you can stroke the insides of her thighs. Use that feather-light touch all the time—or a firm and gentle caress. Move her legs around a bit so you can reach the inside of her knees. Draw little circles with your fingertips around the inside of her knees as you continue to stroke her thighs.

By this time she should be giving you some soft moans and '*mmm*' sounds to let you know she likes what you are doing. This would be a good time for her to give you some guidance if she wants something a little different.

BREASTS

As you feel her body starting to respond, and if she is ready, deepen your kisses, using your tongue to tickle her lips and her tongue. As your kissing gets more passionate, you can start stroking and caressing her breasts. Put your palm over her nipple and think of energy flowing out of your palm into her nipple. Then take her nipple between your thumb and forefinger and gently roll it back and forth. As one nipple hardens in arousal, you can move to the other nipple and make sure it gets its fair share of attention. Again, she should be making some kind of noise to let you know she likes what you are doing. This is a good time to suck on her nipples and draw them into your mouth, licking and sucking them. Suck on one nipple while manually teasing the other, rolling it between your thumb and forefinger.

You may notice that her nipples are firmer toward the tip. That's the most sensitive part. The area just behind it, the areole, has nerve endings as well. Try using your index finger, middle finger, and thumb to gently squeeze this area and stroke out to the end of the nipple. If you are sucking, you can bite very gently on the nipple. Think of rolling a grape between your teeth and not breaking the skin of the grape.

VULVA

Once you have aroused her nipples, you may want to keep sucking on one of them while you let your hand move down to her pubic area. If she has one knee up with the foot on the bed, that will open her crotch and make her genitals more accessible. Using that ultra-light touch, stroke that hollow between her thigh and her labia. You can cup her whole genital region in your hand and gently massage it. Try pulling gently on the pubic hair just above her clitoris. This will pull on the clitoral hood and in turn stimulate her clitoris.

Split your fingers so you can gently massage up and down on either side of her labia minora. Notice if there is any fluid present on her labia. If there isn't, use some of your saliva to lubricate her labia and begin to stroke slowly up and down. It's important that these sensitive tissues be well lubricated.

CLITORIS

After some of that stroking, begin to focus your attention on her clitoris. Using the moisture from her vagina and your saliva, begin to circle around her clitoris, again using a very light touch. Her labia needs to be very wet and slippery. If they are not, USE LUBE! Make it a practice to keep lube close by whenever you are making love.

Everything in her vulva should be slippery by now. You can slide your fingers on either side of the clitoris and rub up and down. As you feel the labia and the clitoris swell in erection, that indicates her level of arousal is getting higher. Using your fingers, stretch the clitoral hood back to expose the glans. The clitoral hood is much like the foreskin on the penis that covers the glans of the penis.

For many women, the most sensitive area on the clitoral glans is about the one to two o'clock position as you are looking straight on at her genitals. Because it is so sensitive, always be sure that there is plenty of moisture or lube when you touch the glans. You can occasionally dip your fingers into her vagina to bring out more lubricant or use more saliva.

Never put anything dry in a dry vagina, not a finger or penis or anything else.

It's almost always a good idea to use lube.

PASSION

By this time, she should be aroused. If her hips are moving, and she is thrusting with her hips, she's turned on. It's like that song, "The Hips Don't Lie." If you're not sure, ask her. If she's really ready, she could be begging you to come inside her or to give her an orgasm.

By this time you should be so turned on that you can't wait to get inside her. Let her know how passionate you feel and that you want to ravage her, in a loving way of course. Now would be a good time to move into The-Play.

Ladies, if you've had enough Fore-Play let him know. If he's not reading your signals, say something like, "I need you inside me, NOW!" or "Lick me NOW!"

Before you leave this chapter, there are a few more things to keep in mind about Fore-Play.

WOMEN'S EROGENOUS ZONES

There are different areas of women's erogenous zones, and there is an order in which you should approach them. Remember earlier, how I said no two women are alike? So bringing a technique that was learned from one woman may not work at all on a different woman.

There are some things that seem to apply to many women, but an important thing to know is her 'hot buttons,' her erogenous zones, and to understand that what touches arouse her can change from day to day.

It's always a good practice to ask a woman what turns her on and then do that. That doesn't mean you can't also try new things. Create a practice session where you try the items on the list in Appendix III and remember her response to each one. For each subsequent encounter, you can try or add more of them and see how she responds. In another session, you may reverse the practice and have her try things on you and see how you respond, and how she responds to doing it. If you have the audio version of the book, you can play it and I will lead you through the exercise.

It might also be a good idea to go over that list with her at some time when you are not making love. Ask her what she likes and what she doesn't like on that list.

Here are some things to keep in mind as you develop your Fore-Play.

An important thing to understand is that women get erections much like men do. The clitoral system extends deep into her body and becomes engorged and swollen like a penis. (See Anatomy in Appendix I).

LUBRICATION

Some women self-lubricate a lot and others hardly at all. In later life, during peri-menopause or post-menopause, women generally have less moisture in their vaginas unless they are taking some kind of hormone replacement. (You'll find an excellent discussion about this in the Sex After Fifty chapter). Make sure your woman is wet enough to take your penis without any discomfort.

Just because a woman's vagina is wet doesn't necessarily mean she is aroused. Wetness is an automatic protection response. Check with her to be sure.

Saliva can be good to get started but will dry out if not replenished or supplemented with a lubricant. Note also that some women do not like saliva on them at all; ask and find out! Most couples use water-based lube available on the Internet or in the drug store. It's a good idea to stay away from the flavored, scented lubricants and an even better idea to check out what you are using with a Google search for toxicity and ph balance.

As I mentioned, every woman is different, and there are some women who actually don't want lengthy foreplay. The key is communication. You have to pay attention to how she is responding and listen to what she says. Ladies; if you're not getting what you like, you have to tell him in words, or if nothing else grab him and put him where you want him. He'll go along with you.

FORE-PLAY FOR A MAN

As I mentioned earlier, men do not need much foreplay, but here are a few things to know:

Doing a strip tease dance will almost always turn him on.

Many men like to have their nipples played with.

Fondling his penis and scrotum is very sensual and exciting; especially if oral sex is not the main event, then that is an excellent way to get him erect.

Having him lying on his back as you straddle his face and play with yourself or while he licks you is very exciting for some men. Touching and stroking all over his body excites almost all men. Dangling your breasts over his mouth with your nipples just touching his lips is a great tease.

If you are feeling kinky, you can tie his hands over his head then tie his ankles together and play with him. You could also blindfold him. However, since men are so visual, it might be a bigger turn on if he watches you naked as you play with him. And he might like to be spanked, tied up or not.

Ask first!

BONDAGE

Let's get a little kinky for a minute. There is an element of sex play that includes Pre-Play and Fore-Play, and that is bondage. Bondage play can be very sensual and freeing. I'm not talking about sadism, just sensual restraint.

You may want to go a little further in the BDSM game. To be sure you know, BDSM stands for Bondage and Discipline, Dominance and Submission, Sadism and Masochism. We are only interested in the bondage and discipline parts—however, that does imply some dominance and submission. One person is the top, and the other is the bottom. One does the tying, and the other is tied. You get the idea. We want this bondage scene to be romantic and sensual—and consensual.

MAKE AGREEMENTS

Fifty Shades of Grey, or Anne Rice's *Sleeping Beauty Trilogy*, turned on millions of enthusiastic women because many of them had fantasies of being restrained and passive while being forced to have ecstatic orgasms. A lot of them would masturbate to these fantasies. The key word here is fantasy. Women really don't want to be forced, they only want the illusion of being forced in a safe and consensual way. This is what we call "Romantic Bondage."

It's a good idea to talk things over so that you both have something of an understanding of what you are going to do. It's also a good idea to agree on a 'safe word' to use in case it gets too uncomfortable for her. The reason to use a safe word is two-fold. It provides a clear communication to stop whatever is happening. Some use the "green, yellow, red" words to mean, "Green means go ahead, Yellow means slow down and let's talk about this, and Red means stop immediately."

Another thing to decide is who is going to be in control. Who will be the dominant and who will be the submissive? It's okay to take turns.

SET THE STAGE

Where do you want to play? In the bedroom, or is there another place that you can trick out into your "Fungeon"? Some people set things up in the basement, some use the garage; apartment dwellers have to be even more creative. Wherever you set up, make it clean and attractive.

One way to have access to your partner's body for lots of teasing and caressing or some light flogging, is to use one of those over-the-door hooks so that your partner has her arms held up and away from her body. You can also put eye bolts at each corner of the bed so that you can tie your partner spread-eagled to the bed. There are some straps to put under the mattress that you can order on-line that will do the job as well.

Another part of setting the stage is the lighting. Make it soft and warm. Use candles when appropriate. Don't make it too dark because the visual effects are part of the whole scenario. You might want to create a playlist for your games as well: music always adds a nice touch.

COSTUMES

For me, costumes are a big part of the game. Seeing my partner in a shelf bra and thigh high stocking and those spike heels is a huge turn on. There are things for me to wear as well. It's fun to look through the online catalogs and pick out things you both might like.

BONDAGE PLAY

The first thing to say is that it's not a good idea to restrain someone with ropes unless you're experienced in rope play. The ropes can cut off circulation and may be difficult to untie in the event of an emergency. The same can be said for scarves and neck ties. It's best to use some Velcro bondage cuffs which can easily be obtained from Amazon and a combination of snap latches and cord which you can get at the local hardware store. The Velcro cuffs can be quickly released and will still provide the feeling of restraint that you are looking for here. Some even have a synthetic fur lining to make them even more comfortable.

Once your partner is in restraint, all the elements of foreplay we discussed will work. A sleep-mask blindfold adds another element to the arousal. If you really want to get kinky, you might also use some soft leather whips to tease and titillate. There are some multi-strand floggers made out of suede or deerskin that make a lot of noise when they strike but don't really hurt when they are used with care. It would be a good idea to look at some of these whips at an adult toy store before investing.

I have always considered B&D games as a part of foreplay. Sometimes having a woman tied up and lightly teased is just the thing to bring her focus into the present moment so she can truly enjoy the sensations that will titillate her and enable her to have a fantastic orgasm. Something about being restrained makes the sensations even more exciting.

If the scenario that you set up is not conducive to actually having intercourse, simply unclip your sweetie and move the action to the bed where you will probably not bother with the bondage because you are so hot to get into each other.

Play the way you have agreed to play and check with your partner periodically to see if everything is okay, and have fun with it. I don't mean to imply that you have to make bondage a part of your Fore-Play every time. It's just something you can do on occasion if you wish.

SPIRITUAL SEX

To have magical sex, you want to raise the level of excitement and arousal. That leads to high energy and high vibrations, which cascade into a release of endorphins, norepinephrine and dopamine. This triggers a response in the right pre-frontal cortex, which is the same area that lights up when one is having a spiritual experience. And that's magical.

However you do Fore-Play, do it in a way that will bring you both to the highest possible level of arousal. The higher the arousal the greater the magic. Keep that passion strong as you move into The-Play.

CHAPTER SIX

Step 3: The-Play

Okay, I know we're getting close to the climax, but this is a good time to take a little break and get a clear picture of what we're dealing with here. Take a look at these illustrations so you know what you are doing and how it impacts arousal.

To begin with, let's identify things by their real names.

- *The vulva* means all the external female genitals.

- *The mons* is the area over the pubic bone, usually covered with pubic hair, and

- *The vagina* is the tube-like canal where the penis (or fingers, toys, etc.) goes in and the baby comes out.

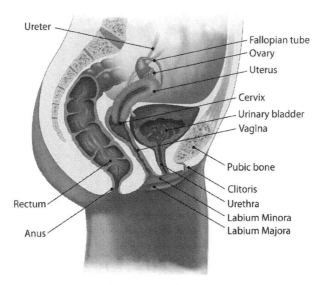

Figure 1 (illustration credit: Kacakayaali)

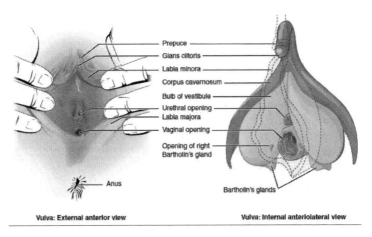

Figure 2: Wikipedia: illustration from Anatomy & Physiology, Connexions website. http://cnx.org/content/col11496/1.6/, Jun 19, 2013.

There is a much more detailed description in Appendix 1. Now we can talk about The-Play.

ORAL SEX

Orgasms are usually the most intense sexual energy a woman experiences. The more powerful the orgasm, the greater the magic. That's why oral sex really does count as sex! Oral sex is a very important part of magical sex, because as we mentioned, somewhere between fifty and eighty percent of women do not orgasm from vaginal sex. Most women need direct clitoral stimulation to achieve orgasms.

Therefore, it is a good idea to know how to make oral sex exquisite for your partner. So, our "ladies first" policy applies here too, as we want to make sure that she has an opportunity for an orgasm before we do.

But first...

Maybe you've heard of the Australian kiss? It's like a French kiss, but down under.

CUNNILINGUS: ORAL SEX ON A WOMAN

Some women need as much foreplay for oral sex as they do for intercourse and some do not. Here is another situation where the teaching tools we talked about in chapter two come into play. Almost every woman has a different way that she likes to receive oral or manual sex, and it can change from day to day. Some women don't like cunnilingus at all, and others just want to get to penetration as soon as possible.

I want to remind you that with fertile women, those who are pre-menopausal, the zones that are most erogenous for her can change from day to day because of the hormonal fluctuations in her menstrual cycle. What worked on one day may be irritating on the next day.

Confusing? Well, maybe a little, but once you get to know your partner well, you will see if she is affected by hormonal changes. But also, livening things up with variety just keeps things spicy and fun! And there's nothing wrong with that, is there?

The key for you is to stay present and keep your focus. Read her cues, and if you're not sure if what you are doing is working, *ask*. However, some women—just like some men—have a difficult time talking when highly aroused. Work together to develop certain moans, grunts, and groans—or even a cue word—to indicate that she likes or dislikes what you are doing. Pay attention to her breathing and the movement of her hips, observing what causes her strongest responses and then staying with it. Women: telegraph what you like and don't like with your body language, whisper to us, even confide in us afterward what you wish we would do next time. We cannot read your mind, but with your help we can learn to read your body, and we welcome simple spoken guidance and clarification along the way. Trust us, it is not anti-sexy!

CUNNILINGUS SCENARIO

Let's continue with our story of what this lovemaking can look like.

You've done enough Fore-Play to be sure she is thoroughly aroused, and now you are ready to take her to the realm of magic. Here's how things can progress from here.

You're in the bed, her hips are moving, and she is moaning, and she wants you *now*. Your kisses are deep and passionate. You're fondling her breasts and teasing her nipples. Taking your time, you kiss your way down to her vulva. You take a pillow and slide it under her hips to raise her up enough so that you don't have to strain your neck. Her legs are spread, she is wide open, and you are ready to start "dining at the Y." Kiss up and down her thighs. Blow softly on her open labia. Put more little kisses and licks in that hollow between her thighs and her labia.

Begin to lick her swollen labia minora, soft, gentle licks going slowly up and down each side of her labia as you work your way to putting your soft tongue into her vaginal opening.

After a few licks there, tease your way up to the U-spot, where the labia minora come together, just above the urethra. Now use your tongue to gently flick the clitoral hood from side to side, and then you can very gently suck the whole clitoris into your mouth. Pay attention to her response to your sucking to make sure it's pleasurable for her.

NIPPLE PLAY

At some point, you can reach around her legs and take her nipples between your thumb and forefinger and roll them gently. For many women, there is a strong connection between her nipples and her pelvic nerves, which will arouse her even further.

FOCUS ON THE CLIT

Once you have her clitoris in your mouth, gently suck it in and then flick the underside of your tongue back and forth over that sensitive nub. Use a sucking in and out action on her clit as you continue to lick it with the underside of your tongue. If she likes a firmer stimulation, cover your teeth with your lips and nibble gently on her clit.

Now, take note again: women are different! The clitoris of some women is so sensitive it can't take direct stimulation. If you're not sure again, ask. If she does have a sensitive clitoris, then keep your stimulation on the hood, and don't pull it back to expose the glans.

To expose the clitoral glans, take one hand and put it on her mons, over her pubic bone, and pull upward gently to stretch the hood back off the clitoral glans.

Continue to lick side to side with the underside of your tongue.

USE A FINGER

When she is responding to your licking, you can bring one hand back around so that you can slip your finger into her vagina. Just up to the first knuckle to begin with and then as she opens up more you can push in a little further. You can let some of your saliva flow down to the vaginal opening before you slip you finger into it. Some women may not be comfortable with that, so ask her if she likes what you are doing. If she does like it...

Continue to lick and suck, rotate your finger around in her vaginal opening. As you do that, you will stimulate the legs (known as the crura) of her clitoris and the vestibular bulbs, all of which will heighten her arousal.

G SPOT

Before we continue, we have to take a break and pause to unravel the mysteries of the G spot. The idea of the "G" spot is somewhat misleading because it's not really a spot, it's an area. It is the spongy tissue that surrounds the urethra; the tube that runs from the bladder around the pubic bone and ends at the urethral opening just above the vaginal opening. See the Figure below. This spongy erectile tissue only becomes erect and apparent when a woman is aroused. Like an erect penis.

If you put your finger all the way into her vagina, and move it from the eleven o'clock position to the one o'clock position, all the way around her pubic bone, you will feel the swollen urethral sponge and its soft uneven ridges. There may be one spot on that spongy surface that is more responsive than others and that could be called the "G" spot.

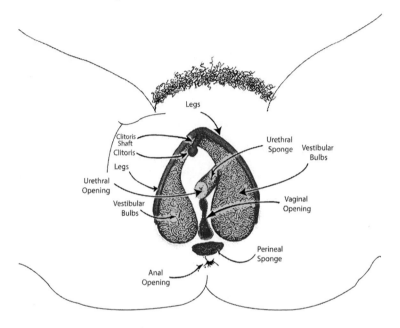

Figure 3 (© Sheri Winston. IntimateArtsCenter.com)

CONTINUING CUNNILINGUS

Now you can take it off pause and hit play as we resume our oral experience.

As you continue to suck and lick, start moving your finger in and out. As your finger goes all the way in, curl it up around her pubic bone and then move it back and forth like a windshield wiper.

Another area that could be responsive is the perineal sponge. The area between the vaginal opening and the anus. You can massage this area when you have your index finger in her vagina, you can use the knuckle of your middle finger to press on her perineum.

If she wants you to go even further with this finger stimulation, you can let the saliva run down past her perineum. Wet your middle finger or little finger with that saliva and begin to rim her anus. After stimulating her anus, you can slip one of those fingers into her anus and then move your hand so that both fingers are sliding in and out of their respective orifices.

If you do put a finger in her anus, be sure that you don't get that finger near her vagina without first washing it off as you can introduce damaging bacteria to her vagina.

Most women can achieve orgasm after somewhere between fifteen and forty-five minutes of this stimulation. The time it takes usually depends on how well you did the Pre-Play and Fore-Play. It's usually about twenty minutes. If she gives you directions during this, do it the way she wants it done.

Then you should be hearing things like, "Oh yeah, don't stop, keep doing that," or "More, yes," or maybe she just moans and pants or holds a hand on your head to keep you there.

BREATH CONNECTION

Breath is the primary energy you need to live. Yoginis have taught Pranayama for centuries. *Prana* means "vital life force," *yama* means "control." Mystic practitioners teach that you can channel that energy by focusing on where you send the breath. Advanced sexual practitioners will tell you that breath plays an important part in getting the most from your sexual energy.

What you want to know is how to use the breath to have magical orgasms. Here's what we were taught in Tantra and you can do this while giving her oral sex.

To keep you focused and connected to her, as you breathe in, visualize her sexual energy coming through her clitoris, which you are sucking on. Feel that energy coming into your mouth and then into your heart.

As you exhale, send that energy back from your heart and out of your mouth onto her clitoris. She will feel this energy exchange, and it will take her higher. To give it more power, as you are exhaling, clench your PC muscles (the muscle use you to stop urinating) and feel that energy coming all the way up from your sex, through your heart, out your mouth, and into her. When you inhale her energy, your level of arousal will also expand and you will feel a deeper connection to her.

At this point, there are two ways you can go as a couple. You can keep licking and sucking until she has an orgasm, or you can move into intercourse.

REACHING ORGASM

If you are going for her orgasm, once she begins to orgasm, just keep doing whatever you were doing. She is depending on the rhythm you have established to get her to orgasm. Don't speed up or slow down and don't start asking her questions about your technique! It will just bring her right down again and you'll have to start all over.

Don't go harder or softer. Just keep doing exactly what you were doing as she started to orgasm. And keep doing it until she asks you to stop.

Many women can have very long orgasms or go from one orgasm into another. At some point, her clitoris may get so sensitive, any more stimulation could be painful, and so if she asks you to stop or pushes your head away, you can stop.

And now you are creating magical sex. All that sexual energy that you helped her generate is bathing both your souls and lifting you higher.

FELLATIO: ORAL SEX FOR MEN

If you are going for intercourse and your erection has diminished, you may want to try fellatio, commonly known as a blow job. Remember the old saw: "Suck, honey; blow is just an expression." Fellatio is best performed with the doer between the legs of the receiver, whether he is standing, sitting, or lying down.

Here are a few factoids about blow jobs you may already know, but she may not, so you can pass this on or read it together.

The penile shaft doesn't have as many nerve endings, so it doesn't respond to licking very well. It does respond nicely to pressure. Squeezing the shaft with the hand, (or the vagina, in intercourse) feels extremely good. Many men can get hard just by squeezing the shaft of the penis.

FELLATIO SCENARIO

To continue our narrative, here's what she might do…

She might start by taking the head of your cock into her mouth and slowly licking around the foreskin, or the glans, depending on whether you are circumcised. Once she has enough saliva on your cock, she can pull the foreskin back and take the head of your cock into her mouth. Then she can lick the frenulum, just under the coronal glans. This is a very sensitive area and should have you moaning with pleasure very quickly.

As she continues to suck and lick, she can take your cock deeper into her mouth and get the whole thing wet. Then she can begin to use her hands on your shaft while she continues to lick and suck the glans and frenulum. The shaft does respond to pressure and friction, but most of the nerve endings are in the glans and the frenulum.

Here's a little trick that may help: have her cup your scrotum in her hand and wrap her thumb and forefinger around the scrotum, above your balls. She can pull down gently on your scrotum, not squeezing the balls, to pull the skin further away from the glans. Then using her lips, she can pop the head in and out of her mouth and the sensations on the rim of the glans are exquisite.

Another little trick is to have her massage your perineum, the area between the scrotum and the anus. This is a very sensitive area for many men. And of course she can slip a finger into your anus, which is also full of nerve endings and responds well to stimulation.

Just as every woman is different, so are men. Men also have those nine nerve endings that terminate in different places in the pelvic area. Experiment with different techniques, and guys, don't be afraid to ask for what you want.

By now, you should be ready for penis-in-vagina intercourse.

PARTNER INTERCOURSE

If you just finished going down on her, you may want to start out in the missionary position. It's simple to move up so you are kneeling between her legs, and you can rub your cock over her labia and clitoris, teasing her and making sure she is wet enough for penetration.

If she is not, or if you're unsure, use lube; it's always best to use more lube than not enough, and you cannot really have "too much" lube. Now that she is wet and ready, start by just inserting your cock head enough to have your coronal glans go just past her vaginal sphincter and then come back out, but keep the tip in contact with her vaginal opening. Do this head-popping a few times and then begin to go deeper with each stroke.

As you start to reach full penetration, move up so you are supporting yourself on your elbows. You can kiss her and look into her eyes, making that deep loving connection. Begin to synchronize your breathing with her, inhaling on the out stroke and exhaling on the in stroke. When you are in all the way, you may want to rotate your hips, so the head of your cock makes a circle inside her vagina. This may stimulate her cervix—try it out and see, slowly, as some women find it uncomfortable; again, no two women are the same. Some women may have nerve ending on their cervix that respond to that stimulation and others may not. You can also grind on her pubic bone, which may stimulate her clitoris.

When you were giving her oral sex, notice how close her clitoris is to her vaginal opening. If it's close, you may be able to get the shaft of your penis to rub against her clitoris.

Experiment and talk about it as you practice.

Be conscious of setting up a rhythm with your breathing and your stroking. Continue kissing while paying attention to your breathing.

That rhythm gives her something she can build on to possibly reach a vaginal, or "G" spot, orgasm. You can try the classic, nine shallow and one deep, or nine deep and one shallow. Try head-popping on the shallow strokes and hip rotation on the deep strokes.

If you don't want to stay in the missionary position too long, you can just roll over while you are still coupled and do the woman astride, "cowgirl" style.

If she has been giving you head while you are lying on the bed, she can come up and straddle you and slowly sit back on your cock. That way, she can control the penetration, which might make the entry more comfortable for her.

WOMAN ASTRIDE

I especially love the woman-astride position. It means you don't have to use energy holding yourself up so you're not crushing her, as in the missionary position. Your hands are now free to caress her, play with her nipples, squeeze her bottom, and finger her anus, she can rub her clitoris while you play with her nipples. She can control the sensations and the rhythm which can also help bring her to orgasm.

Many women like to use their fingers to stimulate their clitoris while riding astride their man. Some use a vibrator instead of fingers. If this brings her to a higher level of arousal and orgasm, so much the better.

If she lays her chest on your chest, you can kiss as you are making love.

USING THE BREATH TO CIRCULATE ENERGY

During this kissing, you can reach amazing levels of ecstasy. As you have your cock inside her, and your tongue kissing her tongue, you are creating a powerful circuit of energy.

You inhale on the outstroke and exhale on the in stroke. As you exhale, visualize the loving energy coming from your heart, down your spine and out your cock into her vagina.

She then takes that energy and brings it up to her heart, and then up to her mouth where you are connected by your tongues.

Then take the energy from her mouth into your mouth and down to your heart. This synchronized breathing will create a closeness and bonding that leads to the limbic resonance we discussed earlier.

The outstroke can be very shallow, just enough to keep friction on the penis and keep it nicely hard. With this pattern, you can stay in a state of bliss and ecstasy for a long time. This is not "deeper, harder, faster" porn sex, just the opposite.

Slow, loving, connected sex that will lead to magic.

At some point, you may need to speed up and go harder and faster to get the stimulation you need to get to orgasm. You can still keep the connection and feel the presence of your lover as she channels her energy into you.

She's had her orgasm and now that you've had your orgasm, don't be in a hurry to get up or clean up. Just lie there and get your breath. Be conscious of the loving energy you have created. Then you can move into After-Play. But before we leave The-Play, let's discuss some things you can do to keep variety in your lovemaking.

VARIETY

If you trained yourself as I suggested in Men's Orgasm Training, you can put that to good use now and have multiple orgasms while connected to your lover. Think of how much sexual energy you will be creating and sharing.

Next, you will probably want to make love in a couple of different positions just to keep things interesting. Doggy-style can provide interesting sensations for both of you. You feel her pelvic bones hitting you just over your pubic bone, and there are a lot of sensory nerve endings there. She might like that angle for the way it hits her internal hot spots. Experiment and keep communicating about what feels good or not so good. Woman astride and facing away can also give some different sensations for you both.

By the way, the idea of mutual, simultaneous orgasms is not necessary to have magical sex. Simultaneous orgasms can happen, and it may be something you want to try for, but it may take a bit of training and practice for a couple to be able to do it on a repeatable basis.

Okay! Now it's time for After-Play and Sex Magick.

CHAPTER 7

Step 4: After-Play

DEEPENING THE LOVING CONNECTION

Now you're both basking in post-orgasmic glow. You have both generated a lot of oxytocin, the bonding hormone, especially during orgasm. This means that she is feeling very connected to you and wants to cuddle with you and savor the contented ecstasy she is experiencing.

Depending on how you created the energy during your lovemaking, you are either fully charged or you want to go to sleep. If you want to snooze, it might be because you have just released a huge amount of energy, emotional charge, or stress, and are totally relaxed and comfortable. For now, just experience what's happening for you both.

Men release the greatest amount of oxytocin they ever experience when they climax, so you'd want to cuddle too, right? Wrong, because right after orgasm men get a big shot of testosterone too.

Guess what? The testosterone blocks the oxytocin. So instead of wanting to cuddle, you probably feel like you want to get up and do something, like getting something to eat, or watching TV. Cool your jets. Take fifteen or twenty minutes to be with her and let her know how much you love connecting to her like this and what it means to you.

You can do this non-verbally just by stroking and caressing her as she lies next to you.

I like it when I'm lying on my back and my wife puts her head on my shoulder, and puts her leg over so it rests on my crotch. I can reach around her with one arm and stroke her head or her back and use the other arm to caress her arms.

This is not the place for wham-bam-thankyou-ma'am. Now is the time to cherish her and bond with her on an even deeper level. Consciously creating a loving closure to your sexual intimacy is an important step for magical sex. Think of it as a continuing investment in your relationship, happiness and joy.

SEX MAGICK

There's a lot of woo-woo and hoo-doo around Sex Magick, so take what you like and leave the rest. You can have fun and play with it.

To give you some historical perspective, Sex Magick has been performed by spiritual traditions since time immemorial. I was told that it has its roots in pre-historic Shamanism, which is hard to prove. I was, however, first introduced to it by a Native American

Shaman forty years ago. There is historical evidence that shows it was carried out in ancient Egypt and Babylonia. Both Hinduism and Buddhism have tantric yoga sects that have practiced it for centuries and continue to this day. In modern times, there are neo-tantric groups worldwide that that have embraced it.

THE LAW OF ATTRACTION

Currently, the concept of the Law of Attraction has gained great popularity. It states that our thoughts have energy and what we think of is what we tend to attract. The more positive our energy when we direct our thoughts towards the outcome we desire, the more powerfully we draw, like a magnet, the results we want. Sex Magick is basically an application of that understanding.

We know that sex has energy, and the energy is highest at the moment of orgasm and shortly thereafter. The idea of Sex Magick is to combine the energy of the orgasm with our thoughts, thus supercharging their attractive power.

Kaballah, the mystical branch of Judaism, been teaching this for thousands of years. After climax, couples unselfishly focus their thoughts outward for the blessing, healing, and benefit of others and the world.

Sex Magick works best and has most power when you have a clear and exact vision of what you want to manifest. That means you can actually see yourself having whatever it is you want to be, do or have. Feel the emotion. How will you feel when you have it? If you say, "I *want* XYZ," you are affirming the lack of XYZ. Instead think, "I *have* XYZ." Judith and I usually do this right after we climax, but if we haven't, we do it while we're snuggling.

Remember, this doesn't mean that you just sit around waiting for delivery of your dreams. Powerful intention and focused action creates the reality you desire.

SEX MAGICK CEREMONY

I'm certain that there are many ceremonies from many traditions that I will never know, but I can share a few things I learned from some very esoteric teachers. Use what you like or modify the ceremonies to make it work for you. And of course, make it fun.

Some teachers recommend that you create a little altar near your bed. On it, they suggest you put something that represents the four elements: earth, air, fire and water. Candles can be a part of it. Incense is also good.

If you really want to get fancy, get a piece of red paper and cut it into a triangle. Write whatever it is you want to manifest on the paper and put it on the altar with the point of the triangle aimed at you in the bed.

After your orgasm and after you've focused your thoughts on what you desire and are ready to get up, take the red paper with your desire written on it, and smear some body fluids from your lovemaking onto to the red paper.

Burn the paper in the sink and wash it down the drain as you release your vision into the universe. Then forget about it and let the universe bring it to you as you take whatever action is needed to manifest your dream.

CREATE A SIGIL

Other teachers emphasize the importance of creating a sigil, which is a symbol that is thought to have magical powers. You can create your own sigil. Make a list of all the things or states you want to manifest and create the sigil that represents what you desire. The sigil will plant those things you desire in your subconscious and speed up their manifestations.

Here are some ideas to give you an example of how to create a sigil.

Let's say you want more love and intimacy in your life. You could use the classic symbol of a heart to represent love and intimacy.

Maybe you also want to have more loving sex so you might write the word SEX inside the heart symbol.

If you want to manifest more money, you can put the dollar sign $ inside the heart as well.

To top it all off, you visualize having good health and you can use something like a red cross or a Caduceus and put that over the top of everything else.

It might look like a jumbled mess (or a work of art) to anyone but you. However, you know what it means and what it represents. Plant those ideas in your subconscious. You can keep the sigil on your altar or put it on the red triangle, or you could put it up in various places in your home and have it remind your subconscious of what you desire.

In the past, I have used this whole ceremonial process that I just described, with excellent results. Other times we both simply spoke out loud the things we wanted to manifest, and had good results that way as well. Our focused high-vibration thoughts have attracted the goodness we seek in our finances and our creative endeavors, often from unexpected sources. It doesn't cost anything, so why not give it a try? Great sex often comes from trying out new things.

CHAPTER 8

Sex After Fifty

Nearly 40% of the population in the USA is over fifty - which means that a lot of us are dealing with the effects of menopause and andropause. Of course, everything in the previous chapters about sex applies to seniors as well, but there are some additional factors to take into account as a result of aging.

ABOUT MEN OVER FIFTY

Men experience a change of life that's much less pronounced than what many women experience in menopause. In fact, many men aren't consciously aware that it's happening until one morning they wake up and say, "What happened? Where did my sex drive go? Why do I feel depressed?"

WHAT IS ANDROPAUSE?

Andropause, sometimes called "male menopause," is the result of the natural, slow, steady decline of testosterone (T). After the age of thirty, T starts to decrease by 1%-2% a year, so that by the time a man is fifty-five, he has 25%-50% less; at sixty-five, 35%-60% less; etc. Depending on how much T he was genetically endowed with and the percentage that is decreasing, he is impacted to a greater or lesser degree.

So everything that T supports will be reduced to a greater or lesser degree due to andropause, including a man's sex drive, energy, and self-confidence. This is when a guy can have more difficulty getting and maintaining erections, may feel more fatigued, can lose muscle mass. A guy can develop an enlarged prostate, and even have hot flashes and night sweats.

Depressing, for sure.

There's more: emotionally, a man can feel anxious, experience mood swings, a bad temper, irritability, feel burned out, and have less drive or ambition. Does that sound like the 'grumpy old man' syndrome?

And he probably thinks that everyone *else* has the bad attitude.

To make things worse, his estrogen is increasing. A startling little-known fact is that the average fifty-four-year-old man has higher estrogen levels than his fifty-nine-year-old female counterpart! (That is, unless she's taking hormone replacement therapy and her estrogen is about the same as pre-menopause.)

This estrogen leads to more belly fat, which as we know is difficult to get rid of. Another thing is, being a little overweight and eating carbs generates aromatase, a substance that creates the undesirable chemical reaction of converting some of his diminishing testosterone into estrogen, which leads to more belly fat. All this tends to make a man sensitive about his appearance and his libido.

Wow. What's a guy to do?

PARTNER SUPPORT

Ladies, if you're in a relationship with one of these guys, you can tell him how much you care about him and ask him how you can support him in cleaning up his act. Encourage him to reduce his carbs, get his T levels checked and maybe set up some kind of exercise program that will help him get things going. At least two-and-a-half hours of exercise a week seems to be the magic number. Going for walks together is a great way to start.

I know men are so resistant to changing anything, or taking advice from a woman who starts to sound like "Mom." But give it shot. Give him this book. Maybe it will work. Getting him to make those changes will make his (and your) life better and make him strong and sexy again.

If his doctor indicates he has low testosterone even after these changes in diet and exercise (healthy sleep habits help too), you may want to encourage him to consider testosterone replacement therapy (TRT).

One thing to know about TRT is that once you start on it, you may be pretty much stuck with it, because you stop making your own testosterone. But practically speaking, if it's already low and getting lower by the day, your body won't ever be able to make enough anyway.

It's pretty common these days to do TRT and there are plenty of different ways to do it: patches, gels, a buccal patch on your upper gum, injections, and subcutaneous pellets which your doctor inserts under your skin every three to six months. Each method has its pros and cons, so your doctor will have to figure out which is best for you. My doctor likes injections, because the gel is subject to losing potency at higher temperatures, and the oral version goes through the liver, which isn't a good thing.

My T levels got so low, I finally elected to do it.

Am I glad I did!

Now I'm physically stronger, my mood is good, and my libido is back.

LOW, OR NO, SEXUAL DESIRE

For many of us, when we hit a certain age, we seem to lose our desire to have sex. We think about it occasionally, and would like to have that physical release we remember as being so pleasurable, but the drive isn't there.

What Judith and I found is that your desire will follows your arousal. So if you get naked and do the things you each like to do, you'll get aroused and feel desire. As I said before, suit up and show up and the game is on. Touching, skin to skin, will generate oxytocin. That bonding hormone will help you connect to her, and oxytocin will flow from the brain, down the spinal column, and come out in the pelvic nerve endings, helping you to get and sustain an erection.

So, make a date and show up with a willingness to play.

SEX

Remember how I said women generate oxytocin by talking, and great communication is what most turns a woman on? Generally, testosterone blocks oxytocin, so when you were younger you probably didn't necessarily want to talk a lot and maybe you weren't that great at being intimate.

The good news is that being a mature lover can give you the gift of finding more satisfaction through deeper intimacy. Without all that T blocking your oxytocin, you can enjoy cuddling, taking your time with a lot of kissing and touching, and holding each other more. The closeness you feel might be a revelation; plus, this is the kind of connection she's always wanted with you.

Even if the oxytocin is flowing and your bonding is wonderful, you may still have problems with your erection. In that case, use oral and manual techniques to give her satisfaction and by that time, you may become sufficiently aroused by seeing how turned on she is. Generic versions of Viagra and Cialis are readily available. The pills work for most men, so it's definitely worth a try.

Sometimes, your partner may be satisfied with the sensual erotic experience she is having, and whether you penetrate probably isn't that important. As mentioned earlier, most women have clitoral orgasms anyway and if the woman is menopausal, her vaginal dryness may be a problem.

Another issue that can become a concern is fatigue. As a man ages, he may not be able to hold himself up for very long in the missionary position. Many men find it easier to be on their back with the woman on top. This way, you can both coordinate your movements to get the most stimulation, and this position is also good because it frees up your hands so that you can caress and stimulate her.

Having said this, some women also find the 'woman on top' position tiring or may find it hurts their legs. So, the bottom line is that you need to work as a couple—and talk lots—to find out the best senior sex positions that work for both of you.

After fifty, a sufficiently firm bed and some good pillows definitely helps. If she's on top, you can put a firm pillow under your buttocks to raise you up and pillows under each of her legs to make her comfortable. If she's on the bottom, you can put the pillow under her buttocks to raise her up and position pillows under her widespread, bent knees to make her open and relaxed. I hear that yoga blocks can help too, but only if there's a pretty firm surface under them.

COMMON MALE ISSUES THAT CAN BE RESOLVED

Some things I've learned when talking to men in this age bracket is that they want sex and they can get an erection, sometimes with the help of Viagra, Cialis, or something like that, but a couple of factors keep them from having a satisfying sexual experience.

The first factor is that, as men age, it may take a longer period of stimulation to reach orgasm than it used to. It's the opposite of premature ejaculation. Like the old joke, "It takes me all night to do what I used to do all night." This leads to the second factor, which is they run out of energy before they get to the finish.

They've done the Pre-Play and Fore-Play and feel deeply connected to their partner. They may perform cunnilingus until their partner has her orgasm. This has them excited and erect, and they get started with intercourse, and when their energy runs out, so does their erection.

Some guys ask their partner to give them oral and manual sex until they orgasm. Another man told me that he loves to perform cunnilingus on his partner while he masturbates. She kneels over his face so that he can lick her while he masturbates. After his orgasm they snuggle in After-Play using Sex Magick to create the things they want in their lives.

If a man wants to have an orgasm while connected and inside his partner's vagina, they can adapt their practice so that he gets that orgasm while his energy level is good and then make sure to give her an orgasm, when his energy returns. That way they can both have a satisfying, magical sexual experience.

Others told me that they can get hard and orgasm while looking at porn, but when it comes to having intercourse with their wife, nothing works. The good news is that they can get it up and get it off, the bad news is multi-layered.

Looking at porn usually means looking at beautiful young bodies. That conditions the subconscious to respond to those same kinds of images, so when the man looks at his older wife, he may not be inspired in the same way. This could also cause her to feel that her body isn't attractive enough and in effect constrains her desire for him, because she feels inadequate.

As we know, as a man ages, he has less and less sexual energy available to him. If he is dissipating that sexual energy by masturbating to porn, it stands to reason that he will have less sexual energy to give to his partner when they want to make love. Therefore, it might be a good idea for him to stay away from masturbating to porn for two to four weeks and see if he has more sexual energy for her.

Another problem is when a guy really wants to have sex and satisfy his partner but can't sustain the energy to have the kind of sex he used to have. His desire to perform becomes a burden on him, and when he doesn't perform or have the kind of pleasure he wants, he gets frustrated or depressed; being triggered, of course, can prevent him from climaxing, even if he's masturbating with her beside him. This negative self-fulfilling pattern impedes his future sexual encounters. As you might imagine, the negativity is contagious; his partner's concern about his attitude dampens her libido too, so sex becomes a problem for her as well. Not much fun. Then, perhaps for other emotional reasons, one or the other partner may not really want to have sex.

Resolving this and every other problem will take time and willingness from both partners to have non-judgmental discussions about their sexual challenges and feelings. These discussions have to be done in a safe, caring way. The goal is to work out how to create a loving, fulfilling, and satisfying sexual connection with each other.

The key in all of this is open and honest communication. I suggest you go back to the section in Chapter Two, Communication For Lovers, and re-read the section called "Beginning the Conversation" together.

He may have fantasies that he wants to fulfill with her that he has never even mentioned to her, for fear of rejection. She may be experiencing vaginal discomfort as a result of peri-menopause or post menopause that she has never mentioned to him, because she wants to please him. Everything should be discussed. That doesn't mean each partner has to fulfill every fantasy the other one has, but at least they can talk about it, to see if there is some way to be accommodating.

If having this conversation is too difficult or upsetting for either of you, it might be a good idea to seek the services of a love, sex, and relationship coach. Resolving old hurts and unfulfilling experiences can open the door for a new and revitalized sex life.

You've come this far, don't stop now.

ABOUT WOMEN OVER FIFTY

WHAT IS MENOPAUSE?

It's important to understand the woman you're dealing with has probably gone through some important physical, emotional and mental changes as a result of her change of life too. There are phases, and each has a name, so let's define them.

Menopause is the day twelve months after a woman stops getting her period. That's it. Her body is irrevocably altered: no more eggs; minimal ovarian output of sex hormones. *Post-menopause* is every day after that, her new "normal" for the rest of her life.

What leads up to the day her menses stand still is *peri-menopause*. Unlike T, women's hormones don't have that regular orderly march down to lower levels. As her ovaries slow down, her estrogen (E) and progesterone production can become completely unpredictable, causing hormonal imbalances which affect her body, emotions, and mind. This transitional time usually starts in her forties, but can begin as early as her late thirties or after her mid-fifties. It can last two to ten years. And you thought you had problems!

Both peri-and post-menopause affect every woman differently. She may or may not have various symptoms, including: hot sweats;

mood swings; anxiety or depression; anger; forgetfulness; thinning hair; weight gain; problems sleeping and fatigue.

Sexual issues can be a big one.

Just as your lower T and higher E makes you more mellow, her lower E makes her less mellow. Post-menopause, a woman's proportion of T to her E can be as much as twenty times higher than it was in her fertile years. Consequently, she can become more aggressive, adventurous, independent, risk-taking, goal-oriented, and focused on getting what she wants—all characteristics of high T. The one area that's not a given with the preponderance of T is an increased sex drive and ability to experience pleasure.

WILL SHE WANT SEX?

It depends. As in all things, the 'every woman is different' rule applies. Although some women still have a healthy drive, and others feel more pleasure than ever, a great many have problems.

Let's start with the bad news first. That way we can end with some happy good news.

Both during peri-menopause and later in post-menopause, a woman can experience bloating; tender breasts; dry skin; vaginal dryness; vaginal itchiness or burning; thinning of her vaginal wall; painful intercourse as a result of the last two points; a diminished sexual response and diminished sexual pleasure; and decreased desire for sex.

It's not a given that she'll have sexual difficulties. Some lucky ten to twenty percent of women just breeze through perimenopause and others just have mild symptoms. Not everyone has the same symptoms or combination of symptoms.

Although we haven't found statistics on sexual issues in perimenopause, we have found studies on post-menopause. The American College of Obstetricians and Gynecologists found that 87% of married post-menopausal women in their study experienced decreased desire, 83% had difficulty climaxing, 74% had poor lubrication, and 71% felt discomfort when they made love.

Other studies found that 25%-45% of postmenopausal women found sex painful, mostly due to vaginal dryness. 93% of the women who said they were in pain still had intercourse, and 40% made love once a week or more. *Ouch.*

Of those, 73% of them only did it to please their partner.

Many women in the survey were too embarrassed to talk to their lovers about their vaginal and sexual symptoms. What's more startling is they were also too self-conscious to tell their health professionals.

That's just sad.

It is crystal clear that you need to create a safe space and initiate a frank discussion with your partner about what's going on with her emotionally and sexually. You need to ask questions, listen, and accept the answers. No blame, no "what about me?" You've got to understand the problems in order to work as team to find the solutions.

Vaginal dryness is a major culprit in making sex a turnoff for women. It both hurts to have sex and it increases the risk of getting vaginal, urinary tract, and bladder infections. Dry conditions create a two-pronged threat: firstly, estrogen withdrawal causes a woman's genital tissue to thin and shrink. When it thins down to a single cell, it can get microscopic tears, especially when you enter; secondly, vaginal fluid needs estrogen to maintain its acidity, and without it, bacteria thrive. Those microscopic tears enable bacteria to get into her body and travel up to her urethra and bladder, leading to uncomfortable and even dangerous infections.

WHAT CAN YOU DO?

It's really important to support her in finding a remedy to vaginal dryness in particular and peri- and post-menopausal symptoms in general. There are many products that help women with their symptoms. She doesn't need to suffer.

To relieve atrophy and dryness, there are low-dose prescription estrogen inserts, as well as natural moisturizing gels.

HORMONE REPLACEMENT THERAPY

For overall well-being, there is *hormone replacement therapy (HRT)* and *bio-identical hormone replacement therapy (BHRT)*, both of which replace her E and progesterone (the latter is needed to prevent uterine cancer.)

HRT products are patented, FDA approved, chemically altered or completely synthetic hormones. Bioidentical hormones are extracted from plants and prepared in the labs to have exactly the same chemical and molecular structure as the hormones the body produces. The commercial ones are FDA-approved.

There are all kinds of hormone replacement delivery options, including: a patch, tablet, capsule, lozenge, sub-lingual drops, gel, vaginal cream, vaginal insert, vaginal tablet, suppository, skin cream, and spray.

It's up to her to study the pros and cons of hormone replacement, and if she goes for it, her doctor will help her choose which one best suits her needs.

If she's not interested in hormone replacement, a lot of alternative or integrated doctors also use herbs and natural medicines to help with peri- and post-menopausal symptoms.

Judith has used the bio-identical estrogen and progesterone transdermal creams since peri-menopause and credits them with helping her maintain a good personal and sexual quality of life.

HER LOW LIBIDO

The same advice I had about your own low libido and desire applies here. Set aside a time to lie in bed. Take your time in Pre-Play and Fore-Play. Talk to her, communicate, stroke her, kiss her, and connect with her. Once the oxytocin kicks in, desire comes with it and leads to a very satisfactory and pleasurable experience. It's the old 'fake it till you make it' trick.

THE GOOD NEWS

For the passionate women of post-menopause who naturally have a healthy sex drive as well as those on HRT or BHRT, being post-menopause frees up their energy. No PMS, cramps and monthly bleeding, no contraceptives and worrying about pregnancy. If they've had kids and they are out of the house, there's finally time and space to explore their sexuality undisturbed.

Their experience and confidence pay off in bed. Unlike the ladies who feel it's taboo to discuss their needs, these sensualists of "a certain age" ask for what they want. So be prepared to up the ante. A woman might also have reached the point where she's more experimental and adventurous.

If your mate's libido is alive and well, you could have the added pleasure of seeing her have more orgasms and multi-orgasms than she had before menopause.

In terms of tips for better sex, everything in the previous chapters applies to senior sex as well. I worked at sex until I became proficient and knowledgeable about my own sexuality, sex in general, and my wife's sexuality in particular. I did it and I'm now in my mid-eighties, still doing it. Don't hold back.

If you want to find out a lot more about sex in general, andropause and menopause, I again strongly urge you to go to Amazon and buy our book, *So THAT'S Why They Do That! Men Women and Their Hormones*. Knowledge is power. We learned so much while writing it that we improved our own sex lives!

Anatomy

At first, I wasn't going to include an anatomy chapter, but as I dug deeper in my research, I learned some interesting things that could best be explained using anatomy diagrams. In addition, as I wrote, I realized that it would be helpful to see the diagrams to better understand exactly what you're dealing with. Some things you might learn could be the key to taking her—and you—to a higher level of arousal. And we all want that.

FEMALE ANATOMY — SECRETS OF HER LADY PARTS

You might have looked a lot of genital diagrams or seen a lot of "pussies" and "cocks" on erotic web sites. Even so, please do yourself and your partner a huge favor and take a closer look at these diagrams. To begin with, let's identify things by their real names.

- *The vulva* means all the external genitals.

- *The mons* is the area over the pubic bone, usually covered with pubic hair, and

- *The vagina* is the tube-like canal where the penis (or fingers, toys, etc.) go in and the baby comes out.

Some men—and women too, actually—wrongly use the word vagina when they really mean vulva. Not all the female genitals can legitimately be called a vagina, no matter how much we might like to call it that.

So now you know.

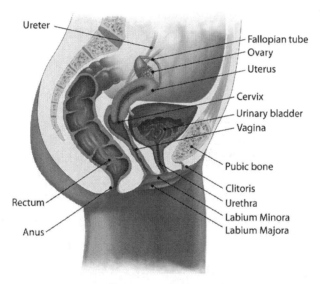

Figure 1 (illustration credit: Kacakayaali)

The *labia majora*, the outer labia, help keep the vulva closed and protect the more sensitive inner labia, the labia minora. As a woman becomes aroused, the labia majora shrink and allow the labia minora to be exposed. What's interesting to note is that the vestibular bulbs are located (Figure 2) behind the labia majora and when you cup a woman's vulva and massage it gently, you are stimulating the vestibular bulbs.

The *labia minora* help protect the vagina. The labia minora can vary a lot in color, size, and shape, and no two women are alike. As a woman gets aroused, these labia fill with blood and get erect, much like a penis. These sensitive labia minora need to be kept wet whenever they are being touched and can heighten arousal and lubrication when they are gently fondled or stroked.

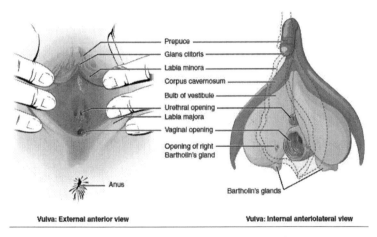

Figure 2: Wikipedia: lustration from Anatomy & Physiology, Connexions website. http://cnx.org/content/col11496/1.6/, Jun 19, 2013.

THE CLITORIS

The *clitoris* sits at the top of the labia minora. It's covered by a fold of skin called the *clitoral hood, or prepuce,* much like the foreskin of an uncircumcised penis. Under the clitoral hood lie the *clitoral shaft and clitoral glans.* In Figure 2, you can see the whole clitoral system. There are over 15,000 nerve endings in this system, over half (8,000) in the clitoral glans. The purpose of the clitoral system is to give pleasure to the woman. She really likes that, and we do too. By giving pleasure via the clitoral system, the woman self-lubricates more, easing the way for smoother penetration, and this enhances the facility to become pregnant in child-bearing years.

The clitoral shaft under the hood can be rubbed and stroked, as long as it is kept moist. The hood and shaft can take more and longer stimulation than the very sensitive glans. Once the woman is completely aroused, you can put a finger on her mons and gently stretch the hood up to reveal the glans. Very light stroking and licking can provide an exquisite sensation that will often lead to orgasm. Some women are especially sensitive in the one to two o'clock position on the glans, and for a few, it may be too much. Therefore, if the woman is too sensitive for this kind of direct glans contact, try gently rubbing the hood in that same magic spot—one to two o'clock.

G SPOT

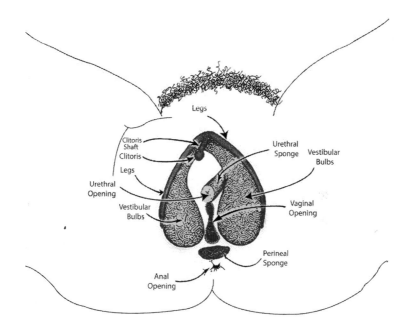

Figure 3 (© Sheri Winston. IntimateArtsCenter.com)

The idea of the "G" spot is somewhat misleading because it's not really a spot, it's an area. It is the spongy tissue that surrounds the urethra; the tube that runs from the bladder around the pubic bone and ends at the opening just above the vaginal opening. (Figure 3)

This spongy erectile tissue only becomes erect and apparent when a woman is aroused. Like an erect penis. You can feel it on the roof of her vagina once she is aroused. If you move your finger back and forth from the eleven o'clock to the one o'clock positions inside her vagina, all the way in and around her pubic bone, when she is aroused, you can feel the soft uneven surface of the area. There may be one spot on that spongy surface that is more responsive than others and that could be called the "G" spot.

Massaging that spot can lead to an orgasm. Put your finger all the way in the vagina and curve it upward in a come hither motion, and you will feel the urethral sponge over the pubic bone. You can also use a side-to-side motion like a windshield wiper along the urethral sponge, or use an in-and-out motion to find out what feels best for her.

BARTHOLIN'S GLANDS

Just inside the labia minora are *Bartholin's glands,* which provide the lubrication for the vaginal area. We like that. You'd never see the tiny openings that leak the fluid, unless you had a light and magnifying glass to locate them.

THE VAGINA

The *vagina* is the birth canal and the intercourse canal.

It normally is collapsed but can expand enough for a baby's head to pass through. In normal sexual activities, it can accommodate most sized penises with proper arousal. The average depth of an unaroused vagina is 3.77 inches, expanding to about seven inches when aroused. Much bigger penises can be painful. The vagina can tent, that is, expand widely when aroused. However, a large penis or sex toy can still be painful and cause damage if used improperly.

THE CERVIX AND FORNIX

At the end of the vagina is the *cervix,* which is where the sperm goes to fertilize the egg. The area just around the tip of the cervix is called the *fornix* (Figure 1). The area toward the front of her body is called the *anterior fornix.* Some researchers claim that stimulating the anterior fornix can generate more vaginal lubricant and be very pleasurable as well. It's been called the "A" spot.

Some women can orgasm from stimulation in these areas as well.

THE PERINEUM AND ANUS

The area between the vagina and the anus is the perineum. This spongy area also expands as a woman becomes aroused and erect. Many women have sensitive nerve endings in this area, and it responds to massage just as it can in men.

The last area to discuss is the anus. There are many wonderful nerve endings in the anus and most men and women will respond pleasurably to light anal penetration and stimulation. You may want to put a lubricated finger in the anus to stimulate all those nerves, as a part of foreplay or during intercourse. You can also use a dildo, a butt plug or your penis. Some women can orgasm during anal intercourse.

PELVIC NERVE ENDINGS

A few more comments about women's genitalia.

There are nine pelvic nerve endings from the brain to the pelvic area. They don't go to the same places on every woman, though. As we mentioned, no two women are alike. That's why in addition to clitoral orgasms, some women can have cervical orgasms, some have 'G' spot orgasms, "A" spot orgasms, anal orgasms and others. The sensitivity can vary from day to day. And wonderfully—it's all normal!

WOMEN'S ORGASMS

Much has been written about women's orgasms. We mention some types of orgasms, and other researchers have listed eleven types of female orgasms. What most agree on is that the biggest factor in women having an orgasm starts in her brain. That's why Pre-Play is so important.

The best way for women to explore her orgasmic potential is to masturbate and try using vibrators or dildos to find out what works best for her.

On average, it takes a woman about 20 minutes of stimulation to reach orgasm. Most women's orgasm can last from 13 to 51 seconds, and she can have multiple orgasms. Men's orgasm only lasts from 10 to 30 seconds, and men have to wait for a period before they can have another orgasm.

MALE ANATOMY — HOW TO GET HIS MAGIC WAND TO MAKE MAGIC

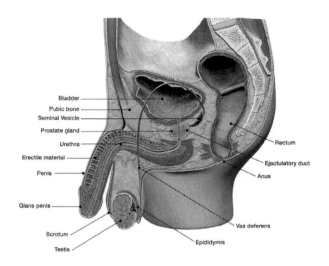

Figure 4 (illustration credit: Hank Grebe)

EXTERIOR GENITALIA

The *penis* has chambers called the corpus cavernosum, which fill with blood to make the penis erect. A study published in the British Journal of Urology in 2015 found the average length of an erect penis was a little more than five inches.

The *glans,* the bulb at the end of the penis, is home to about 6,000 nerve endings; that makes it the most sensitive part of the penis. The area under the head of the penis is called the *frenulum.*

The frenulum and the foreskin are also very sensitive and filled with nerve endings, so respond very well to light touch and licking.

The shaft of the penis has fewer nerve endings and responds more to squeezing than light stroking or licking.

The perineum is the area between the scrotum and the anus and massaging it feels very pleasurable. Some men really enjoy anal stimulation and you can insert a lubricated finger to bring more pleasure.

INTERIOR ELEMENTS

The *vas deferens* is a tube that connects the sperm-producing testicles to the ejaculatory duct. When men get a vasectomy, that tube is either cut or tied off, preventing sperm from leaving the testicles, and it's a very effective form of birth control. (I had a vasectomy 45 years ago, and it hasn't affected me adversely at all). The vas deferens joins the ejaculatory duct just above the prostate, and after the seminal vesicles.

The *prostate gland* secretes fluid that helps boost the volume of the semen, and its smooth muscles contract, causing the semen to ejaculate.

This walnut-sized gland can cause lots of problems for men as they get older. Getting prostate massage regularly may contribute to long-term prostate health, and some men also find prostate massage very arousing, so it's worth exploring.

Get yourself some latex gloves and lube, and have your sweetie give you a prostate massage. You might like it and she might enjoy having her fingers inside you, instead of it always being your fingers inside her. Of course, it's a very good idea to have things cleaned out in there before playing.

The *seminal vesicles* sit just above the prostate and can be massaged through the anus. Often, when massaging the prostate, semen leaks out and some of that comes from the seminal vesicles.

You'd probably never even know about these little guys, but if they weren't there, you'd definitely miss them. *Cowper's glands* are responsible for the pre-cum that leaks out of the penis during arousal. The pre-cum neutralizes the acidity in the urinary tract before the sperm cells are ejaculated.

So, there you have it, boys and girls. That wasn't painful at all,

Step 1: Pre-Play Exercises

PHYSICAL EXERCISES THAT BRING YOU INTO THE MOMENT

Now that you've read the chapter on Pre-Play, here are some playful things you can do that will lift you to an even higher level of magical sex.

A lot of sexual/spiritual teachers advocate doing body movement prior to sex, because it gets your blood flowing and energy up. We have some recommended exercises below, but anything that gets you moving, present, and bonded, works. Is there some exercise you like to do together? Biking? Running? Tennis? Hiking? Yoga? Do it and have fun. When you've finished you might want to come home and shower together, and then go to the bed and do the sitting exercises.

After movement, sitting exercises are recommended by sexual/spiritual teachers because they open up your internal channels so that your sexual energy flows freely throughout your body, heightening your connection to your lover, responsiveness and experience. It's play, so give it a try, and get your spirit self and your physical self present in the moment.

You might like to do these exercises naked, by the bed. You can do them in the order listed or you can mix and match, doing whatever brings you the most fun and energy.

HIP THRUST

Many of us have very little motion in our hips. This exercise will loosen those hips up.

- Stand feet shoulder width apart, knees bent slightly.

- As you inhale, clench your PC muscle (the muscle you use to stop peeing) and thrust your hips back.

- As you exhale, release the clench and thrust your hips forward.

- As you get comfortable with this exercise, you can add the sound "Ha" when you thrust your hips forward.

Do this for 1-2 minutes.

ECSTATIC DANCE

Create a music playlist that has a powerful drum beat that goes on for at least five minutes. Maybe it's R&B, maybe rock and roll, whatever you like. After the drum beat music, add a couple of slow dance tunes that will last another five minutes.

Start the music and let your bodies move independently for at least five minutes. If you're into it, you can do it as long as you like. After the ecstatic dance come together for a slow dance. This is not ball room dancing. It's more like hugging and swaying to the music. Maybe your thighs are intertwined and you're rubbing together.

A fun addition is to whisper sexily in each other's ear in a language that you make up as you go. You'd be surprised how much sensuality your playful invented language can convey.

After dancing, move to the bed for the next series of exercises.

SPIRITUAL EXERCISES TO CONNECT YOU TO YOUR LOVER

EYE GAZING

Looking into someone's eyes for a period of time is a powerful and intimate practice that creates an opportunity for deep emotional connection. When you are focusing on each other's "window to the soul," you are both exposing yourselves and receiving each other. The vulnerability might feel a little uncomfortable at first, but you will be creating a sense of safety and bonding because direct prolonged eye contacts stimulate oxytocin, the bonding hormone.

Like all the exercises, the goal is to be completely present with your lover. When you are here, now, you and your whole body are sensitized, and your ability to taste, touch, hear, see and feel her and every delicious thing is tremendously magnified.

But sitting and gazing into someone's eyes can be challenging. Our thoughts can distract us. Sometimes our bodies don't feel good or we suddenly feel like we're going to nod off. Don't worry. It can take a while to get present. If you realize your thoughts are wandering or you are going unconscious, just put your attention back on your lover's eyes. Eventually your focus will get better. Like all exercises it takes training and repetition, but the rewards are great.

Start with shorter periods. You can set a timer and start with thirty seconds at first if you wish. Add a few seconds each time you do it until you get to at least five minutes. You can go longer after that if you want, but five minutes should be enough for you both to feel connected and bonded.

This is a very intimate practice. If your partner is struggling, don't take it personally. They are probably doing their best. Break the gaze, because the idea is to feel good and connected, not overwhelmed.

Talk about what is going on and see if you can make any progress by doing very short gazing intervals.

Here is what to do:

1. Sit comfortably, facing your partner. You can touch or hold hands if you like.

2. Set your timer for the time you wish.

3. Take a deep breath and gaze into your partner's eye. Many teachers recommend you focus your left eye on her left eye because the left eye is considered receptive. You are both opening to receive each other. Others recommend right eye to right eye. See which one works for both of you.

4. Keep your gaze soft.

5. Keep breathing and blink as you need to.

6. If you laugh, cry, squirm or whatever comes up, just do your best to hold the gaze and keep breathing.

7. When the timer goes off, you can break your gaze.

8. If you want, you can finish with a hug.

SYNCHRONIZED BREATHING

After the eye gazing, you can add synchronized breathing. It's very simple. The man observes the woman's breathing and matches it. Breathe in together at the same time, breathe out at the same time.

It's important for the woman to take full deep belly breaths so the man can see and sync with her.

Breathing together connects you, helps your mutual energies resonate in simple, loving way and relaxes you. Scientists have found that couple's heartbeats are often synchronized, anyway, but this makes you conscious of it. As you breathe together, your energies are going back and forth and you really feel each other. A little smile will relax your mind and deepen your absorption.

This is a great tool for intimacy that you can use anytime with your lover. You can do it when you're hugging or cuddling, and it is especially wonderful during sex. You can synchronized your breath before you go to sleep. She lays on top and you match her breath. It's very comforting and a great way to end the day.

HAND-ON-HEART

As you get comfortable with the eye gazing and synchronized breathing, you can combine them with the hand-on-heart exercise. This comforting touch allows a loving transfer of energy between you. As before, the man follows the woman's breath.

1. Each of you place your left hand over your partner's heart. Take your right hand and cover the left hand of your partner. Look into each other's eyes with a smile. Breathe in synch with each other. Let the unspoken love for each other be felt through your connection. Feel your hearts entwine and your souls commune.

2. Take a deep breath together. Bring your breath into your belly and then feel it coming up into your chest, all the way up so that it surrounds your heart. Hold your breath for a second or two, then sniff in a little more air and exhale with an "Aah" sound and release all the tensions in your body. Visualize the love energy flowing into your partner's heart.

3. Repeat three times. Then relax and move to the next exercise.

ALTERNATE BREATHING

After you've done hand-on-heart with the synchronized breath, you can practice it with alternate breathing. As with synchronized breathing, you follow her breath.

1. Start by having your lover exhale through her mouth. As she does so, you inhale her breath through your nose. Then you exhale through the mouth and she breathes it in through the nose: the in breath of one is the outbreath of the other. Back and forth you go, taking each other's loving energies in, and circulating them in your bodies. Keep doing it until it's easy and comfortable.

2. Imagine you are exchanging your love and light when you breathe into her, and accepting her love and light when you inhale her breath.

3. You can also imagine you are giving her all your marvelous male energy and accepting all her rich feminine energy. And vice versa.

Alternate breathing is one of those techniques that can make sex more magical.

In oral sex or intercourse, you can pump love/energy/ passion into your partner on the outbreath. She takes it on the in breath, then sends you her love/energy/passion on the outbreath.

You can also exchange energy when kissing by just alternating your breath through your mouths. You breathe into hers mouth, she receives it and vice versa.

Give it a try. See if it builds your intimacy and enhances your sexual experience.

PC CONTRACTIONS

PC contractions will enliven and strengthen the genital area for both men and women. They increase the blood flow to the genitals, resulting in higher levels of arousal and more intense orgasms. For men, it's also the exercise that, with practice, leads to multiple orgasms. So it's REALLY worth doing.

1. As you inhale a deep breath, clench and hold your PC muscle, (the one you use to stop peeing) and feel a lift in your genitals.

2. Exhale and relax.

3. Again, inhale deeply, clenching the PC muscle as you hold the breath, and hold the clench.

4. Now release the clench and exhale. Again, inhale/clench, hold, and exhale/relax.

5. Continue for about twenty repetitions.

6. Now begin to feel the energy building in your genitals.

7. Visualize this energy as a ball of warm light.

8. As you inhale and clench all the muscles on the floor of the pelvis, feel that energy being pushed up your spine to your heart.

9. As you exhale, relax and let that energy stay in your heart.

10. Continue to breathe this way. Inhale, clench, feel the energy move; then hold, exhale and relax. Continue. Now return to normal breathing.

If a woman's pelvic muscles get strong, she can contract them and stimulate her lover's penis during sex. This works best if she's on top. Either he can lie still, or she can contract when as he pulls back or thrusts into her. Or they can create a rhythm together. The contracting turns her on too!

After doing the PC contractions, when you're ready, begin to caress each other and move into Fore-Play.

Step 2: Fore-Play Techniques

FORE-PLAY TECHNIQUES

This is a list of arousal techniques that have worked on different women at different times.

It's something you can use to get familiar with each other's erogenous zones. It's a good idea to discuss this when you're not in the heat of passion. Talk with her about each of the things listed here and ask her if there are any she doesn't like, and which ones she likes the most. If she's not sure about one of these techniques, ask if she's willing to try it. If not, scratch it off the list.

The next time you are practicing your love-making, go through the list and see how it works for you. If you have the audible version of the book, you can play it and follow along as I describe each technique.

FORE-PLAY FOR WOMEN

Remember, there are two things you need to stimulate on a woman for her to become aroused.

1. Her mind. The most sensitive organ in her body is her brain, and it *must* be engaged for her to respond. Her brain never stops working. Your job is to get her out of her head and into her body.

2. Good conversation will get things started and you can spice it up as you go along. Touch will help get her out of her head and into her body. All this is part of Pre-Play.

Remember: if she is upset or worried, she will not be able to open up and relax for good sex.

Fore-Play is almost always about touch, but that doesn't mean you can't whisper sweet nothings or talk dirty to her. She might like it if you talk dirty. Ask.

HANDS AND ARMS

Wrists/palms. Remember those old-time movies where the lothario kisses the palm of the woman? The reason is there are many sensitive nerve endings in the palm. The same goes for the inside of the wrist. Light kissing and stroking will activate these areas. Inside of elbows. Many nerve endings that respond to a very light touch or kissing on the crease. Put the palm of your hand on her heart center and feel the love flowing into it.

HEAD AND NECK

Nape of neck. Light kisses, nibble with teeth or lips.

Ears. A lot of women don't like sloppy licks in their ears, but they do like very light kisses around the ear. Heavy breathing in her ear is another good technique, a very primitive one. Some ancient texts also recommend pulling gently on the ears. Don't do great big lip-smacking kisses around the ear, since the noise can be annoying.

Kissing is a great way to deepen the connection and get the oxytocin, the bonding hormone, flowing. If you are not sure how to kiss her, put your lips to hers and then mimic the way she is kissing you. Some women need to get connected before they can be open to French kissing. The tongue to tongue contact makes a powerful energy connection.

LEGS AND FEET

Behind the knee. Roll her over on her tummy and stroke the backs of her legs and make little circles around the inside of her knees. Kiss the crease on the back of the knee. This can be a very sensitive area.

Ankles/feet. Light strokes around the ankles may work on some women. Foot massage will work on almost every woman. You may also want to try a little toe sucking.

Inner thighs. One of my favorites. I love the smooth, soft skin of a woman's inner thigh. I love to run the tips of my fingers up and down over this area. She will like it a lot as well. Licking here is also very effective.

The crease between the buttock and the back of the thigh is a sensitive place and responds well to stroking. Squeezing the buttocks and light spanking can also be very arousing. Some women like a fairly strong spanking because it awakens many of the nerve ending in the whole pelvic region. Experiment to see what she likes.

ANUS

There are many nerve endings in the anus. Just make sure it's clean and don't let fingers that have played with the anus play anywhere on the vulva without washing them first. Some like to do analingus, where you lick her anus. It's a great turn on; however, be sure it's very clean, otherwise you can wind up with Giardia, which will make you sick. Be sure you ask first. She may not like it.

BREASTS/NIPPLES

Approach the nipples slowly, stroking around the breasts with a light touch and then gently rolling the nipple between your thumb and forefinger. Trap the nipple between your thumb, forefinger and middle finger and gently draw the nipple out. It should harden and become erect as she becomes more aroused.

Rough pinching and tugging may not be a good idea in the early stages of foreplay, but can be very stimulating when she is completely turned on and approaching orgasm. Sucking the nipples will stimulate oxytocin and send signals to her genitals that will heighten her arousal. Spend a lot of time sucking each nipple. You can use your teeth as though you were holding a grape without breaking its skin.

MONS, VULVA, LABIA, AND CLITORIS

This should be in the final stages of Fore-Play. By now her breath rate should be higher, her hips should be moving, and she should almost be begging you to touch her clitoris. Stroke around her outer labia and the hollows between her vulva and thighs. Put your hand on her mons, that's the area just above her vagina, and pull it up a little or pull gently on her pubic hair. This will pull her clitoral hood up and down on the glans. She might like that. It's much like moving the foreskin up and down on the glans of your penis.

Circle your way around her vagina, teasing your way to her inner labia. If you have worked your way through this list, her vagina should be erect, swollen, and very wet at this point. If not, there may some physical reason why she does not lubricate.

When you pull up on the skin or pubic hair just above the clitoris, it will pull the clitoral hood back and expose the clitoral glans. Many women respond to a very light, feather light, stroking at the one o'clock position directly on the glans. This stroking can lead to orgasm, and that orgasm can be sustained with continued stroking on the glans.

Work your way around the inner labia until you reach the clitoris. You can then stroke the clitoris with a wet finger or your tongue and bring her to an orgasm or just make sure she is wet enough for you to penetrate her with your penis. However, just because a woman's vagina is wet doesn't necessarily mean she is aroused. The wetness can be an automatic protection response. You must check with her to be sure.

When aroused, women get erections much like men do. The clitoral system extends deep into her body and becomes engorged and swollen like a penis. A good indication that she is aroused is when her hips are moving. If she is thrusting with her hips, she's turned on.

Some women lubricate a lot and others hardly at all. In later life, during peri-menopause or post-menopause, women generally have less moisture in their vaginas unless they are taking some kind of hormone replacement. Make sure your woman is wet enough to take your penis without any discomfort.

Most use water-based lube products available on the Internet or in the drug store. Saliva can be good to get started but will dry out if not replenished or supplemented with a lubricant. Plus, many women do not really enjoy saliva and would sooner avoid it and use lube; ask for her preference. Never put anything dry in a dry vagina, not your finger or penis or anything else. It's almost always a good idea to use lube.

FORE-PLAY FOR MEN

A few quick reminders of things that arouse a man:

- Doing a strip tease dance will almost always turn him on.

- Wearing a sexy costume will definitely send a message. Ask him what he likes.

- Many men like to have their nipples played with.

- Fondling his penis and scrotum is very sensual and exciting. Especially if oral sex is not the main event, then that is an excellent way to get him erect.

- Having him lying on his back as you straddle his face and play with yourself or while he licks you is very exciting for some men.

- Touching and stroking all over his body excites almost all men.

- Dangling your breasts over his mouth with your nipples just touching his lips is a great tease.

- If you are feeling kinky, you can tie his hands over his head, then tie his ankles together and play with him. You could also blindfold him. However, since men are so visual it might be a bigger turn on if he watches you naked as you play with him. And of course, he might like to be spanked, tied up or not.

Resources

RELATED STUDIES

Hui Liu, Linda Waite, Shannon Shen, and Donna Wang, "Is Sex Good for Your Health? A National Study on Partnered Sexuality and Cardiovascular Risk Among Older Men and Women," *Journal of Health and Social Behavior*, September 2016.

Hsiu-Chen Yeh 1, Frederick O Lorenz, K A S Wickrama, Rand D Conger, Glen H Elder Jr., "Relationships among sexual satisfaction, marital quality, and marital instability at midlife," *Journal of Family Psychology*. June 2006.

Deborah J. Lightner, MD., "Female Sexual Dysfunction," *Mayo Clinic Proceedings*, July 2002

American College of Obstetricians and Gynecologists Practiced Bulletin 213, April 2011

HELPFUL BOOKS

RELATIONSHIP

The Soulmate Experience, Mali Apple & Jo Dunn, 2011.

The Seven Principles for Making Marriage Work, Gottman, John M., 1999. ·

A General Theory of Love, Lewis, Thomas, MD; Aminin, Fari, MD; Lannon, Richard, MD., 2000.

Hot Monogamy, Patricia Love, 1994.

The Female Brain, Louann Brizendine, 2006.

The Male Brain, Louann Brizendine, 2010.

Why Men Never Remember and Women Never Forget, Marianne J. Legato, 2005.

Passionate Marriage, David Snarch, 1997.

The 5 Languages of Love, Gary Chapman, 1992.

So That's Why They Do That! Men, Women and Their Hormones, Judith Claire, Frank Wiegers 2014

SEXUALITY

Mating in Captivity, Esther Perel, 2006.

Naked at Our Age, Joan Price, 2011.

WOMEN'S SEXUALITY

Women's Anatomy of Arousal, Sheri Winston, 2010.

Come As You Are, Emily Nagoski, 2015.

She Comes First, Ian Kerner, 2004.

Tantra for Erotic Empowerment, Mark A. Michaels, Patricia Johnson, 2008.

Human Sexual Response, William Masters and Virginia Johnson, 1966.

TANTRA

Jewel in the Lotus, Saraswati & Avanisha, 3rd Ed. 2002.

Tantra Bliss, Avanisha 2003.

Tantric Love, Sarita & Geho 2001.

SEX MAGICK

The Shaman Method of Sex Magic, Baba Dez & Kamala Devi, 2008.

Modern Sex Magik, Donald Kraig, 2002.

About the Authors

Happily married love, sex, and relationship coaches Frank Wiegers and Judith Claire have seventy years of combined experience helping men and woman achieve the intimate fulfillment they always dreamed of. They've authored the award-winning book, "*So THAT'S Why They Do That! Men, Women, And Their Hormones*," and created the results-driven online dating course *Seriously Seeking Soulmate*.

Frank Wiegers is a fighter pilot veteran of the Vietnam War and a veteran of the relationship wars. When he decided he didn't want any more wars, he began to study everything he could find about love, sex, and relationship.

Desiring to learn how to create connection, fulfillment, and bliss with his partner, Frank studied with teachers from Europe, India, and the US, including a Native American shaman. He approached his training in love, sex, and relationship with the same dedication and discipline that it took to get three degrees (Law, Aero-Engineering, and Business) and to become a fighter pilot. He completed the Science of Mind Practitioner and Ministerial

Course, the Relationship Coaching Institute Singles and Couples Coaching course, and is licensed by The Relationship Coaching Institute.

Judith Claire is a successful personal, relationship, and career counselor and coach in Los Angeles. For more than four decades she has specialized in counseling members of the film industry, creative thinkers, and professionals with spiritual values, because those reflect her own paths and passions. Judith's spiritual studies and practices integrate both Eastern and Western teachings and techniques, and include tantric yoga, a form of sacred sex. Her lifelong purpose is to assist individuals and couples to achieve their full potential.

Praise for
So THAT'S Why They Do That!
Men, Women, And Their Hormones

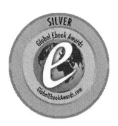

"Nobody in recent memory has written the ABCs and XYZs on the connection between sex, relationships and human hormones in a satisfying way. Claire and Wiegers demystify famously bumpy terrain (fertility, menopause, testosterone, sexual communication) by crafting a clear and comprehensive 21st Century roadmap for the genders. If there is one book to solve World Peace by enlightening couples about their bodies, and solving in and out of the bedroom disputes around the globe, it's *So THAT'S Why They Do That!* Happy landings, indeed!"

– Zaque Gruber, The Huffington Post

"Finally, a user's manual for the opposite sex – and to better understanding yourself when it comes to love and love making. This book distills the wisdom of modern research and practical experience into simple but profound guidelines that will enhance your understanding of the interpersonal dynamics that affect each one of us every day of our lives.

– Jenny Wade, Researcher and author of Transcendent sex:
When Lovemaking Opens The Veil

"*So THAT'S Why They Do That!* is an owner's manual for the human body that reveals how to master your hormones throughout your life to increase romance and happiness. It's the perfect "how to" book for men and women. Everyone will get a kick out of reading it."

– Paul J. Zack, Professor of Ecomoniccs, Management and Psychology at Claremont Graduate University; author of The Moral Molecule: The Source of Love and Prosperity.

"Straightforward and compassionate, this down-to-earth relationship guide explains how hormones act as the silent drivers of behavior for women and men. Of special note is the commentary on unlocking the power of biology to enjoy a lifetime of love and sexual fulfillment, as well as learning communication tactics and understanding methods to resolve conflicts, stay together, and be happy. *So THAT'S Why They Do That! Men, Women And Their Hormones* is exceptionally well informed, impressively presented and very highly recommended."

– The Midwest Book Review

Thanks again for reading our book.

As you can imagine, this book has been an important part of our lives, and we worked hard to make it available to you. When our readers give us a review, it lets us know that the work we are doing means something, and someone appreciated it enough to write about it.

Please help us get this important information to as many people as possible by writing a review of our book. Your review will make such a difference in helping others to get the joy and magic in their lives. We look forward to reading what you have to say.

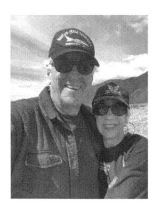

Made in the USA
Middletown, DE
26 February 2022

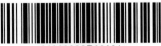

61869989R00091